T0228927

Hospitalization for Heart Failure

Editors

MIHAI GHEORGHIADE
SAVINA NODARI

HEART FAILURE CLINICS

www.heartfailure.theclinics.com

Consulting Editors
MANDEEP R. MEHRA
JAVED BUTLER

Founding Editor
JAGAT NARULA

July 2013 • Volume 9 • Number 3

ELSEVIER

1600 John F. Kennedy Boulevard • Suite 1800 • Philadelphia, Pennsylvania, 19103-2899

http://www.theclinics.com

HEART FAILURE CLINICS Volume 9, Number 3
July 2013 ISSN 1551-7136, ISBN-13: 978-1-4557-7592-7

Editor: Barbara Cohen-Kligerman

© **2013 Elsevier Inc. All rights reserved.**

This periodical and the individual contributions contained in it are protected under copyright by Elsevier, and the following terms and conditions apply to their use:

Photocopying
Single photocopies of single articles may be made for personal use as allowed by national copyright laws. Permission of the Publisher and payment of a fee is required for all other photocopying, including multiple or systematic copying, copying for advertising or promotional purposes, resale, and all forms of document delivery. Special rates are available for educational institutions that wish to make photocopies for non-profit educational classroom use. For information on how to seek permission visit www.elsevier.com/permissions or call: (+44) 1865 843830 (UK)/(+1) 215 239 3804 (USA).

Derivative Works
Subscribers may reproduce tables of contents or prepare lists of articles including abstracts for internal circulation within their institutions. Permission of the Publisher is required for resale or distribution outside the institution. Permission of the Publisher is required for all other derivative works, including compilations and translations (please consult www.elsevier.com/permissions).

Electronic Storage or Usage
Permission of the Publisher is required to store or use electronically any material contained in this periodical, including any article or part of an article (please consult www.elsevier.com/permissions). Except as outlined above, no part of this publication may be reproduced, stored in a retrieval system or transmitted in any form or by any means, electronic, mechanical, photocopying, recording or otherwise, without prior written permission of the Publisher.

Notice
No responsibility is assumed by the Publisher for any injury and/or damage to persons or property as a matter of products liability, negligence or otherwise, or from any use or operation of any methods, products, instructions or ideas contained in the material herein. Because of rapid advances in the medical sciences, in particular, independent verification of diagnoses and drug dosages should be made.

Although all advertising material is expected to conform to ethical (medical) standards, inclusion in this publication does not constitute a guarantee or endorsement of the quality or value of such product or of the claims made of it by its manufacturer.

Heart Failure Clinics (ISSN 1551-7136) is published quarterly by Elsevier Inc., 360 Park Avenue South, New York, NY 10010-1710. Months of publication are January, April, July, and October. Business and editorial offices: 1600 John F. Kennedy Boulevard, Suite 1800, Philadelphia, PA 19103-2899. Periodicals postage paid at New York, NY, and additional mailing offices. Subscription prices are USD 224.00 per year for US individuals, USD 361.00 per year for US institutions, USD 76.00 per year for US students and residents, USD 268.00 per year for Canadian individuals, USD 413.00 per year for Canadian institutions, USD 285.00 per year for international individuals, USD 413.00 per year for international institutions, and USD 96.00 per year for Canadian and foreign students/residents. To receive student and resident rate, orders must be accompanied by name of affiliated institution, date of term, and the *signature* of program/residency coordinator on institution letterhead. Orders will be billed at individual rate until proof of status is received. Foreign air speed delivery is included in all *Clinics* subscription prices. All prices are subject to change without notice. **POSTMASTER:** Send address changes to *Heart Failure Clinics*, Elsevier Health Sciences Division, Subscription Customer Service, 3251 Riverport Lane, Maryland Heights, MO 63043. **Customer Service: 1-800-654-2452 (US and Canada). From outside of the US and Canada, call 314-447-8871. Fax: 314-447-8029. For print support, e-mail: JournalsCustomerService-usa@elsevier.com. For online support, e-mail: JournalsOnlineSupport-usa@elsevier.com.**

Reprints. For copies of 100 or more of articles in this publication, please contact the Commercial Reprints Department, Elsevier Inc., 360 Park Avenue South, New York, NY 10010-1710. Tel.: 212-633-3812; Fax: 212-462-1935; E-mail: reprints@elsevier.com.

Heart Failure Clinics is covered in *MEDLINE/PubMed (Index Medicus)*.

Printed and bound by CPI Group (UK) Ltd, Croydon, CR0 4YY

Transferred to digital print 2012

Contributors

CONSULTING EDITORS

MANDEEP R. MEHRA, MD
Professor of Medicine, Harvard Medical
School; Co-Director, BWH Cardiovascular; and
Executive Director, Center for Advanced Heart
Disease, Brigham and Women's Hospital,
Boston, Massachusetts

JAVED BUTLER, MD, MPH
Professor of Medicine; Director, Heart Failure
Research, Emory University, Atlanta, Georgia

EDITORS

MIHAI GHEORGHIADE, MD, FACC
Professor of Medicine and Surgery, Director
of Experimental Therapeutics, Center for
Cardiovascular Innovation, Northwestern
University Feinberg School of Medicine,
Chicago, Illinois

SAVINA NODARI, MD
Associate Professor of Medicine, Spedali
Civili Hospital of Brescia, University School
of Medicine, Brescia, Italy

AUTHORS

STEFAN D. ANKER, MD, PhD
IRCCS San Raffaele, Center for Clinical and
Basic Research, Rome, Italy; Applied Cachexia
Research, Department of Cardiology, Campus
Virchow Klinikum, Charité – Universitätsmedizin
Berlin, Berlin, Germany

ROBERT O. BONOW, MD, MS
Center for Cardiovascular Innovation,
Northwestern University Feinberg School of
Medicine, Chicago, Illinois

JAVED BUTLER, MD, MPH
Professor of Medicine; Director, Heart Failure
Research, Emory University, Atlanta, Georgia

SEAN P. COLLINS, MD, MSc
Associate Professor, Department of
Emergency Medicine, Vanderbilt University,
Nashville, Tennessee

G. MICHAEL FELKER, MD, MHS
Division of Cardiology, Department of
Medicine, Duke University Medical Center,
Durham, North Carolina

GREGORY J. FERMANN, MD
Associate Professor and Executive Vice
Chairman, Department of Emergency Medicine,
University of Cincinnati, Cincinnati, Ohio

GREGG C. FONAROW, MD, FACC
Professor of Medicine, Director, Division of
Cardiology, Ahmanson-UCLA Cardiomyopathy
Center, Ronald Reagan-UCLA Medical Center,
Los Angeles, California

VASILIKI V. GEORGIOPOULOU, MD
Assistant Professor of Medicine, Division of
Cardiology, Emory Clinical Cardiovascular
Research Institute, Emory University School of
Medicine, Atlanta, Georgia

MIHAI GHEORGHIADE, MD, FACC
Professor of Medicine and Surgery, Director
of Experimental Therapeutics, Center for
Cardiovascular Innovation, Northwestern
University Feinberg School of Medicine,
Chicago, Illinois

MATTHEW E. HARINSTEIN, MD
Heart and Vascular Institute, University of
Pittsburgh Medical Center, Pittsburgh,
Pennsylvania

ANDREAS P. KALOGEROPOULOS, MD, PhD
Assistant Professor of Medicine, Division of
Cardiology, Emory Clinical Cardiovascular
Research Institute, Emory University School of
Medicine, Atlanta, Georgia

BRADLEY P. KNIGHT, MD, FACC
Northwestern University Feinberg School of
Medicine, Chicago, Illinois

STUART KUPFER, MD
Takeda Global Research and Development
Center, Inc., Deerfield, Illinois

MARC K. LAHIRI, MD, FACC
Department of Internal Medicine, Henry Ford
Hospital, Edith and Benson Ford Heart and
Vascular Institute, Detroit, Michigan

CATHERINE N. MARTI, MD
Cardiology Fellow, Division of Cardiology,
Emory Clinical Cardiovascular Research
Institute, Emory University School of Medicine,
Atlanta, Georgia

ROBERT J. MENTZ, MD
Division of Cardiology, Department of
Medicine, Duke University Medical Center,
Durham, North Carolina

MARCO METRA, MD
Cardiology, Department of Medical and
Surgical Specialties, Radiological Sciences
and Public Health, University of Brescia,
Brescia, Italy

FRANK MISSELWITZ, MD, PhD
Bayer HealthCare Pharmaceuticals, Berlin,
Germany

JONATHAN P. PICCINI, MD, MHS
Assistant Professor of Medicine, Division of
Cardiology, Duke Clinical Research Institute,
Duke University Medical Center, Durham,
North Carolina

MITCHELL A. PSOTKA, MD, PhD
Clinical Cardiology Fellow, Department
of Medicine, University of California,
San Francisco, San Francisco, California

TIFFANY RANDOLPH, MD
Fellow in Cardiovascular Diseases, Division of
Cardiology, Duke University Medical Center,
Durham, North Carolina

GIUSEPPE M.C. ROSANO, MD, PhD
Division of Cardiology, IRCC San Raffaele,
Rome, Italy

AMI N. SHAH, MD
Center for Cardiovascular Innovation,
Northwestern University Feinberg School of
Medicine, Chicago, Illinois

ARJUN SHARMA, MD
Career Scientists, Ontario Ministry of Health
and Long-Term Care, Ontario, Canada

SCOTT TAYLOR, RPh, MBA
Geisinger Health System, Danville,
Pennsylvania

**JOHN R. TEERLINK, MD, FACC, FAHA,
FESC, FRCP(UK)**
Professor of Medicine, Section of Cardiology,
San Francisco Veterans Affairs Medical
Center and School of Medicine, University of
California San Francisco, San Francisco,
California

TOBIAS D. TRIPPEL
Department of Cardiology, Campus Virchow
Klinikum, Charité – Universitätsmedizin Berlin,
Berlin, Germany

MUTHIAH VADUGANATHAN, MD, MPH
Resident Physician, Department of Medicine,
Massachusetts General Hospital, Harvard
Medical School, Boston, Massachusetts

STEPHAN VON HAEHLING, MD, PhD
Applied Cachexia Research, Department of
Cardiology, Campus Virchow Klinikum,
Charité – Universitätsmedizin Berlin, Berlin,
Germany

NORMAN C. WANG, MD
Heart and Vascular Institute, University of
Pittsburgh Medical Center, Pittsburgh,
Pennsylvania

Contents

> Annually, more than 1 million patients are hospitalized for heart failure (HF), translating to high healthcare utilization and cost burden. Among patients with hospitalized HF (HHF), approximately 50% have HF with preserved ejection fraction (HFpEF) and 50% have HF with reduced ejection fraction (HFrEF), with the proportion of patients with HFpEF increasing with time. This article defines the epidemiologic landscape of patients with HHF, comparing and contrasting those with HFpEF and HFrEF, and identifies key areas that require further investigation. More complete characterization of these populations may be the first step to developing effective therapies.

> Despite low inpatient mortality and effective symptomatic management, patients hospitalized for heart failure (HHF) experience high postdischarge mortality and rehospitalization rates. HHF represents a widely heterogeneous population with distinct clinical subsets that may require tailored management approaches. Despite this, however, HHF patients are almost uniformly managed with intravenous diuretics, with low uptake of new therapies during hospitalization. This article proposes a practical approach to classifying HHF patients that is focused on guiding individualized inpatient and postdischarge management. HHF is not a single disease but a manifestation of several cardiac and noncardiac processes and thus should be approached as such.

> Hospitalized heart failure (HHF) is associated with unacceptably high postdischarge mortality and rehospitalization rates. This heterogeneous group of patients, however, is still treated with standard, homogenous therapies that are not preventing their rapid deterioration. The costs associated with HHF have added demands from society, government, and payers to improve outcomes. With coordinated and committed efforts in the development of new therapies, improvements may

be seen in outcomes for patients with HHF. This article summarizes concepts in developing therapies for HHF discussed during a multidisciplinary panel at the Heart Failure Society of America's Annual Scientific Meeting, September 2012.

Gregory J. Fermann and Sean P. Collins

Pressure exists to manage patients with acute decompensated heart failure (ADHF) efficiently in the acute-care environment. Although most patients present with worsening of chronic heart failure, some may present with undifferentiated dyspnea and new-onset heart failure. Others have significant comorbidities that complicate both the diagnosis and treatment. The treatment of patients with ADHF is prioritized based on vital signs and presenting phenotype. The risk stratification of patients is the subject of ongoing evaluation. The disposition of patients to areas other than a monitored inpatient bed, such as an emergency department–based observation unit, may prove effective.

Mitchell A. Psotka and John R. Teerlink

Hospitalizations for heart failure (HF) are increasing, and HF is the primary cause of readmission for all Medicare patients. Inpatient HF mortality is poor, but most morbidity and mortality occurs after hospital discharge. Readmissions attributable to HF persist or increase over time after discharge, and past HF admissions predict both readmission and mortality. The heightened risk of readmission dissipates slowly after discharge, suggesting that any intervention should be part of a lasting care package in the outpatient setting. Interventions that apply to multiple common medical comorbidities may be more likely to reduce overall adverse events.

Tiffany Randolph and Jonathan P. Piccini

Improved utilization and optimization of device therapy in the management of patients with decompensated heart failure (HF) is an important clinical priority. Diagnostic cardiac rhythm device data have been shown to predict hospitalization for HF. Cardiac resynchronization therapy is a highly effective therapy for the prevention of HF hospitalization. Evaluation and optimization of cardiac resynchronization therapy should be considered in all patients admitted with HF despite cardiac resynchronization therapy.

Norman C. Wang, Jonathan P. Piccini, Gregg C. Fonarow, Bradley P. Knight, Matthew E. Harinstein, Javed Butler, Marc K. Lahiri, Marco Metra, Muthiah Vaduganathan, and Mihai Gheorghiade

Hospitalization for heart failure (HHF) is commonly associated with symptomatic improvement in response to standard medical therapy, yet there remains a substantial risk of rehospitalization and death. Clinically stable outpatients and decompensated inpatients represent two types of patients with chronic heart failure. In the former, treatment of common heart rhythm disorders with nonpharmacologic electrophysi-ology-based interventions is of substantial benefit in select patients. The potential benefits of these interventions in the hospitalized setting are not well studied. In this review, current knowledge is discussed and future research directions are suggested with nonpharmacologic electrophysiology-based interventions to reduce the morbidity and mortality associated with patients with HHF.

The detrimental pathophysiology of heart failure (HF) leaves room for physiologic and metabolomic concepts that include supplementation of micronutrients and macronutrients in these patients. Hence myocardial energetics and nutrient metabolism may represent relevant treatment targets in HF. This review focuses on the role of nutritive compounds such as lipids, amino acids, antioxidants, and other trace elements in the setting of HF. Supplementation of ferric carboxymaltose improves iron status, functional capacity, and quality of life in HF patients. To close the current gap in evidence further interventional studies investigating the role of micro- and macronutrients are needed in this setting.

The acute heart failure (AHF) population is a heterogeneous group with multiple interrelated noncardiovascular comorbidities. Chronic obstructive pulmonary disease, renal disease, diabetes, sleep apnea, and anemia affect the clinical characteristics and outcomes of patients with AHF and complicate inpatient management. This article summarizes the impact of these noncardiovascular comorbidities in patients with AHF. In some circumstances, careful attention to the diagnosis and management of these conditions in patients with AHF may help to improve patient outcomes.

HEART FAILURE CLINICS

ISSUES OF RELATED INTEREST

Cardiology Clinics May 2013 (Vol. 31, No. 2)
Echocardiography in Diagnosis and Management of Mitral Valve Disease
Judy W. Hung, and Timothy C. Tan, *Editors*
Available at: http://www.cardiology.theclinics.com

Interventional Cardiology Clinics April 2013 (Vol. 2, No. 2)
Saphenous Vein Graft Stenosis and Thrombotic Lesions in Acute Myocardial Infarction
Amar Krishnaswamy, and Samir R. Kapadia, *Editors*
Available at: http://www.cardiacep.theclinics.com

DOWNLOAD
Free App!

Review Articles
THE CLINICS

NOW AVAILABLE FOR YOUR iPhone and iPad

Foreword
A World View of Heart Failure Requiring Hospitalization

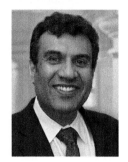
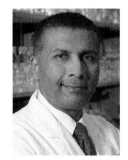

Mandeep R. Mehra, MD   Javed Butler, MD, MPH
Consulting Editors

Disease-modifying therapy with the advent of renin-angiotensin-aldosterone system–directed therapy, β-receptor antagonists, mineralocorticoid receptor antagonists, cardiac resynchronization therapy, and implantable cardiodefibrillators has advanced the natural history of stable chronic heart failure due to low ejection fraction. However, similar advances have remained elusive in the syndrome of decompensated heart failure requiring hospitalization, a heterogenous collection of phenotypic presentations that has failed to produce convincing therapeutic success.

Worldwide, several million hospitalizations for heart failure occur annually with a high burden of recurrent heart failure worsening and deaths of nearly 50% at 6 months after discharge. Arguably, outcomes of stable heart failure (with low ejection fraction) have resulted in lower hospitalization rates but, with the aging of the population and an ever-increasing burden of disease, the cumulative incidence and prevalence of heart failure requiring hospitalization have evolved into epidemic proportions. The economic ramifications of this largely unmitigated disorder cannot be underestimated, and governmental regulatory systems have evolved to discourage readmissions while local administration forces a reduction in length of stay to facilitate use of scarce hospital resources for other higher yield procedures and disease states.

It is interesting to note that during hospitalization, these patients are generally treated with guideline-based recommendations, undergo treatment and control of exacerbating factors, and are presumably provided self-care education for several important aspects. Yet, after discharge, these patients continue to remain at risk for poor short-term outcomes. Several clinical trials have been conducted in hospitalized heart failure patients over the last decade but have not been successful in favorably altering after discharge outcomes. Such therapy, directed to the principle aberrations, has centered on volume control (diuretic regimens and mechanical fluid removal), vascular therapy (vasodilators), inotropic support (catecholamine, inodilator, and myocardial sensitizing agents), and unique neurohormonal therapy (adenosine and vasopressin antagonists). Lessons learned from clinical trials have led to efforts that are beginning to target subpopulations within the vast diversity of presentations as well as use of end points that are clinically meaningful for this unique indication.

Considering these facts, we are pleased to present a dedicated issue of *Heart Failure Clinics* focused on patients hospitalized for heart failure. This issue assimilates up-to-date information in this important field, ranging from epidemiology and pathophysiology to treatment aspects, and provides insight into ongoing

Heart Failure Clin 9 (2013) ix–x
http://dx.doi.org/10.1016/j.hfc.2013.05.004
1551-7136/13/$ – see front matter © 2013 Published by Elsevier Inc.

research directions across worldwide populations with this disorder.

Mandeep R. Mehra, MD
Center for Advanced Heart Disease
Brigham and Women's Hospital
Harvard Medical School
75 Francis Street, A Building, 3rd Floor, Room AB324
Boston, MA 02115, USA

Javed Butler, MD, MPH
Emory Clinical Cardiovascular Research Institute
1462 Clifton Road NE, Suite 504
Atlanta, GA 30322, USA

E-mail addresses:
MMEHRA@partners.org (M.R. Mehra)
javed.butler@emory.edu (J. Butler)

Preface
Hospitalizations for Heart Failure

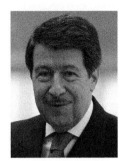

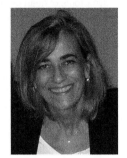

Mihai Gheorghiade, MD   Savina Nodari, MD
Editors

Hospitalization for heart failure (HHF) has been recognized as a distinct entity by regulators and payers only recently.[1,2] It is characterized by worsening of chronic heart failure or heart failure presenting for the first time that requires urgent care. The main reason for HHF is related to severe congestion, manifested by dyspnea and signs of fluid overload rather than a low cardiac output.[1,3] HHF is associated with abnormal hemodynamics, neurohormonal, electrolyte, and renal abnormalities that are rapidly changing during hospitalization and/or soon after discharge.[4]

HHF represents a heterogeneous group that can be divided into those with worsening chronic heart failure (80%), those with de novo heart failure (15%), and those who have advanced or end-stage heart failure (5%). HHF can be further divided into those with preserved or reduced ejection fraction (EF). Distinction should be made between patients with or without coronary artery disease (CAD).[5] The available data from recent registries showed that the mean age of the HHF population is 70 years and, of those, 60% have a history of CAD, 70% have hypertension, 30% to 40% have atrial fibrillation, 40% have diabetes, and 30% have severe renal impairment. The majority of those patient presenting are hypertensive or normotensive,[6] with less than 5% presenting with low blood pressure (BP). The hypertensive response at presentation is related to high sympathetic tone rather than chronic hypertension and is a manifestation of cardiac reserve (the ability to increase BP in response to high filling pressure

and sympathetic tone). In fact, patients presenting with high BP have much lower mortality rates compared to patient presenting with normal or low BP.[6]

Although the majority of patients respond to diuretic therapy and are discharged with minimum signs and symptoms of heart failure and evidence-based therapy consisting of ACE inhibitors/ARBs, β-blockers, and MR antagonists, their post-discharge event rate is unacceptably high (15% and 30% mortality and readmission, respectively, within 60 to 90 days after discharge).[7] This high event rate is seen even in patients who have heart failure with preserved EF.[8] It is important to note that patients who have heart failure with preserved EF represent approximately 50% of entire HHF population and that there is no therapy that has been shown conclusively to affect post-discharge outcomes.

It is alarming that the overall event rate has not changed in HHF patients in the last decade despite the introduction of new therapies for heart failure and implementation of performance measures. In addition, the majority of clinical trials conducted to date were negative in terms of improvement of post-discharge outcomes.[9] This high event rate despite all available therapies makes this topic a health care priority in terms of patient well-being and expenditure. It is possible that aggressive management of congestion, adopting a mechanistic approach to heart failure[10] (find the disease within heart failure), increased utilization of digoxin[11,12] and MR antagonists,[13]

Heart Failure Clin 9 (2013) xi–xii
http://dx.doi.org/10.1016/j.hfc.2013.05.003
1551-7136/13/$ – see front matter © 2013 Elsevier Inc. All rights reserved.

addressing comorbidities[14] such as diabetes and renal abnormalities, judicial use of micronutrients,[15] and an early post discharge visit[16] may reduce the event rate. New therapies[17] should address post-discharge outcome rather than early signs and symptoms during hospitalization.[18,19]

The goal of this issue of *Heart Failure Clinics* is to raise the awareness of heart failure hospitalization as a distinct entity.

We gratefully acknowledge the administrative assistance of Fumiko Inoue.

Mihai Gheorghiade, MD
Center for Cardiovascular Innovation
Northwestern University Feinberg
School of Medicine
645 North Michigan, Suite 1006
Chicago, IL 60601, USA

Savina Nodari, MD
Hospital of Brescia
P.le Spedali Civili 1
Brescia, 25123 Italy

E-mail addresses:
m-gheorghiade@northwestern.edu
(M. Gheorghiade)
savinanodari@gmail.com (S. Nodari)

REFERENCES

1. Gheorghiade M, Vaduganathan M, Fonarow G, et al. Rehospitalization for heart failure: problems and perspectives. J Am Coll Cardiol 2013;61(4):391–403.

2. Vaduganathan M, Bonow RO, Gheorghiade M. Thirty-day readmissions: the clock is ticking. JAMA 2013;309:345–6.

3. Gheorghiade M, Filippatos G, De Luca L, et al. Congestion in acute heart failure syndromes: an essential target of evaluation and treatment. Am J Med 2006;119(12 Suppl 1):S3–10.

4. Gheorghiade M, Pang PS, Ambrosy AP, et al. A comprehensive, longitudinal description of the in-hospital and post-discharge clinical, laboratory, and neurohormonal course of patients with heart failure who die or are re-hospitalized within 90 days: analysis from the EVEREST trial. Heart Fail Rev 2012;17(3):485–509.

5. Flaherty JD, Bax JJ, De Luca L, et al. Acute heart failure syndromes in patients with coronary artery disease early assessment and treatment. J Am Coll Cardiol 2009;53(3):254–63.

6. Gheorghiade M, Abraham WT, Albert NM, et al. Systolic blood pressure at admission, clinical characteristics, and outcomes in patients hospitalized with acute heart failure. JAMA 2006;296(18):2217–26.

7. Ambrosy AP, Pang PS, Khan S, et al. Clinical course and predictive value of congestion during hospitalization in patients admitted for worsening signs and symptoms of heart failure with reduced ejection fraction: findings from the EVEREST trial. Eur Heart J 2013;34(11):835–43.

8. Fonarow GC, Stough WG, Abraham WT, et al. Characteristics, treatments, and outcomes of patients with preserved systolic function hospitalized for heart failure: a report from the OPTIMIZE-HF Registry. J Am Coll Cardiol 2007;50(8):768–77.

9. Gheorghiade M, Adams KF, Cleland JG, et al. Phase III clinical trial end points in acute heart failure syndromes: a virtual roundtable with the Acute Heart Failure Syndromes International Working Group. Am Heart J 2009;157(6):957–70.

10. Gheorghiade M, Pang PS. Acute heart failure syndromes. J Am Coll Cardiol 2009;53(7):557–73.

11. Gheorghiade M, Patel K, Filippatos G, et al. Effect of oral digoxin in high-risk heart failure patients: a pre-specified subgroup analysis of the DIG trial. Eur J Heart Fail 2013;15(5):551–9.

12. Gheorghiade M, Braunwald E. Reconsidering the role for digoxin in the management of acute heart failure syndromes. JAMA 2009;302(19):2146–7.

13. Ambrosy A, Gheorghiade M. Eplerenone reduces risk of cardiovascular death or hospitalisation in heart failure patients with reduced ejection fraction. Evid Based Med 2011;16(4):121–2.

14. Shah SJ, Gheorghiade M. Heart failure with preserved ejection fraction: treat now by treating comorbidities. JAMA 2008;300(4):431–3.

15. Soukoulis V, Dihu JB, Sole M, et al. Micronutrient deficiencies an unmet need in heart failure. J Am Coll Cardiol 2009;54(18):1660–73.

16. Metra M, Gheorghiade M, Bonow RO, et al. Postdischarge assessment after a heart failure hospitalization: the next step forward. Circulation 2010;122(18):1782–5.

17. Butler J, Fonarow GC, Gheorghiade M. Strategies and opportunities for drug development in heart failure. JAMA 2013;309(15):1593–4.

18. Gheorghiade M, Peterson ED. Improving postdischarge outcomes in patients hospitalized for acute heart failure syndromes. JAMA 2011;305(23):2456–7.

19. Gheorghiade M, Braunwald E. Hospitalizations for heart failure in the United States–a sign of hope. JAMA 2011;306(15):1705–6.

Epidemiology of Hospitalized Heart Failure

Differences and Similarities Between Patients with Reduced versus Preserved Ejection Fraction

Muthiah Vaduganathan, MD, MPH[a],
Gregg C. Fonarow, MD[b],*

KEYWORDS

- Acute heart failure • Preserved ejection fraction • Epidemiology • Outcomes

KEY POINTS

- Among patients hospitalized with heart failure (HHF), approximately half have HF with preserved ejection fraction (HFpEF) and half have HF with reduced ejection fraction (HFrEF), with the proportion of patients with HFpEF increasing with time.
- Patients with HFpEF are more likely be women, older, have a history of hypertension, and less likely to have an ischemic cause of HF.
- Although patients with HFpEF may experience lower in-hospital mortality compared with patients with HFrEF, both patients with HFrEF and HFpEF are subject to a similarly high postdischarge mortality and rehospitalization risk.

Close to 6 million patients in the United States have heart failure (HF),[1] with a 25% projected increase in the prevalence by 2030.[2] More than 680,000 new cases of HF are diagnosed each year,[1] which may also be expected to increase as a result of the aging population. The tremendous burden of HF is especially highlighted in the inpatient setting. Roughly 1 million primary and 3 million secondary admissions for HF occur annually in the United States alone.[3] In fact, hospitalization for HF (HHF) represents the leading diagnosis-related group for hospitalizations and rehospitalizations among older adults in this country.[4] These hospitalizations translate to more than 65 million hospital days and billions of dollars of health care expenditures annually.[5]

HHF

HHF represents a potential turning point in the natural history of HF, with these patients experiencing a higher risk compared with patients with outpatient HF (OHF). Since the late 1980s, the drug and device armamentarium for OHF has expanded to include several life-prolonging therapies in patients with reduced left ventricular (LV) ejection fraction (EF).[6] Hospitalization may in itself change the natural history of HF,[7] lending to disease progression and portending marked increases in subsequent event risk.[8] Current national and international guidelines broadly characterize the HF population by EF: HF with reduced EF (HFrEF) and HF with preserved EF (HFpEF). These two HF populations may have distinct epidemiology,

Disclosures: No relevant relationships to disclose (M. Vaduganathan). Research support, Agency for Healthcare Research and Quality (significant); Consultant, Medtronic (modest) and Novartis (significant) (G.C. Fonarow).
[a] Department of Medicine, Massachusetts General Hospital, Harvard Medical School, 55 Fruit Street, GRB 740, Boston, MA 02114, USA; [b] Division of Cardiology, Ahmanson-UCLA Cardiomyopathy Center, Ronald Reagan-UCLA Medical Center, 10833 LeConte Avenue, Room A2-237 CHS, Los Angeles, CA 90095, USA
* Corresponding author.
E-mail address: gfonarow@mednet.ucla.edu

pathophysiology, therapeutic targets, and management approaches. Now, HFpEF, especially in hospitalized patients, lacks clear evidence-based therapies. In order to more clearly define this entity, this article serves to contrast the overall HHF epidemiology in patients with HFrEF and HFpEF.

OVERALL EPIDEMIOLOGIC TRENDS

Certain surveillance metrics of health status have improved for the HF population in the recent past. Length of stay (LOS), in-hospital mortality, and total HF hospitalizations have shown a steady decline over the last decade.[9] Unfortunately, although rates of primary hospitalizations for HF have slightly improved, hospitalizations with HF listed as a secondary diagnosis continue to increase.[3] Despite these advances in in-hospital outcomes, rates of postdischarge readmission and mortality remain relatively unchanged and dismally high.[10] Furthermore, there may be distinct age-, sex-, and region-based differences in HF epidemiologic trends,[4] with younger patients and blacks not experiencing comparable declines in these in-hospital parameters.[11]

DEFINING THE POPULATION

EF represents a quantitative measure of LV function that is broadly distributed in unselected HF populations (**Fig. 1**). EF at the time of HF diagnosis serves as an important index that can help classify the HF population. Patients hospitalized with HF have been categorized as having HFrEF and HFpEF. National guidelines have defined the population with HFpEF as clinically diagnosed HF (based on signs and symptoms of HF) in the setting of relatively preserved or preserved HF. Various cut-off points for EF have been used to define the population including more than 40%, more than 45%, or more than 50%. Others have proposed a middle gray zone of patients with HF and borderline preserved EF, although patients with HF and EF of 41% to 49% seem to have clinical characteristics, treatment patterns, and outcomes more similar to HFpEF with EF of 50% or more than patients with HFrEF. The clinical diagnosis of HF may lack accuracy in certain subsets, including the elderly, the frail, and the obese, thus contributing to possible misdiagnosis of HFpEF.[12] Several working groups have proposed additional criteria, including the Echocardiography and Heart Failure Associations of the European Society of Cardiology,[13] who have put forth that these patients must additionally have evidence of normal LV systolic function and evidence of LV diastolic dysfunction.[13]

Because no clinical trials have yet to be completed in hospitalized HFpEF, most of the data regarding this syndrome are derived from inpatient HHF registries.[14–16] Combined, the Acute Decompensated Heart Failure National Registry (ADHERE),[16] Organized Program to Initiate Lifesaving Treatment in Hospitalized Patients With

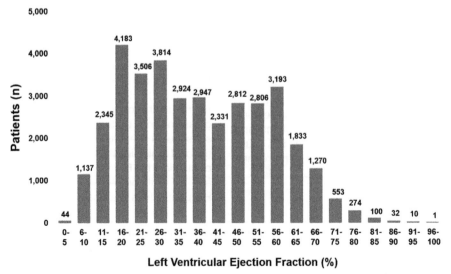

Fig. 1. Distribution of LVEFs in patients hospitalized with the primary discharge diagnosis of HF in the Organized Program to Initiate Lifesaving Treatment in Hospitalized Patients with Heart Failure registry. (*Adapted from* Fonarow GC, Stough WG, Abraham WT, et al. Characteristics, treatments, and outcomes of patients with preserved systolic function hospitalized for heart failure: a report from the OPTIMIZE-HF Registry. J Am Coll Cardiol 2007;50(8):768–77; with permission.)

Heart Failure (OPTIMIZE-HF),[14] and the Get With the Guidelines–Heart Failure (GWTG-HF)[15] registries have reported data from more than 75,000 patients with HFpEF during hospitalization. No established consensus definition of HFpEF currently exists. Regardless of the varying definitions and potential inaccuracies, these studies have revealed a distinct clinical phenotype of HFpEF during hospitalization.

PREVALENCE AND INCIDENCE

Similar to OHF, the relative prevalence of this syndrome during hospitalization seems to be roughly 50%. In 2004, the ADHERE registry estimated a prevalence of HFpEF of 50.4% (EF $\geq$40%).[16] Consistently, in patients with available EF measurements, 51.2% of the OPTIMIZE-HF cohort had EF of 40% or more. Of these patients with HFpEF, 58% had truly preserved EF (>50%), whereas the remaining patients had EF ranging between 40% and 50%.[14] In a slightly more contemporary cohort of patients from 2005 to 2010, 36% of patients had EF greater than 50%, whereas an additional 14% had EF in the borderline range.[15] Across the study time frame, prevalence of HFpEF increased from 33% to 39%, whereas the rates of HFrEF at the time of admission decreased proportionally from 52% to 47%.[15] In 8592 patients in the Prevention of Renal and Vascular End-stage Disease study, the relative incidence of patients with new-onset HFpEF (EF $\geq$50%) was 34% compared with 66% in patients with new-onset HFrEF (EF $\leq$40%).[17]

CLINICAL CHARACTERISTICS

Patients with HFpEF were more likely to be older, women, and less likely to be African American compared with HFrEF. The comorbid disease burden was high in both subgroups; but in general, a history of hypertension and a hypertensive cause of HF were more common in HFpEF.[14–16] Atrial fibrillation and chronic kidney disease may also be more prevalent in patients with HFpEF.[15] Coronary artery disease and an ischemic cause of HF were more commonly noted in HFrEF; prior myocardial infarction was reported in less than a quarter of patients with HFpEF.[16] Most patients had chronic worsening HF (rather than de novo or end-stage HF), with prior histories of HF admissions in approximately two-thirds of patients.[16] Acute pulmonary edema was a rare presentation representing approximately 3% of all patients with HHF.[14] Congestion including dyspnea at rest was generally similar at the time of admission across groups.[15] In terms of vital signs, patients

with HFpEF had higher systolic blood pressures and lower heart rates at the time of presentation.[14] Both cohorts had elevated natriuretic peptides during hospitalization, but patients with HFpEF had significantly lower levels compared with HFrEF.[14] At the time of admission, medication utilization of life-prolonging therapies known to be effective in HFrEF (including angiotensin-converting enzyme [ACE] inhibitors, beta-blockers, and aldosterone antagonists) was less frequently used by patients with HFpEF.[15] Blood pressure–targeting agents, such as angiotensin-receptor blockers (ARB) and amlodipine, were more commonly used by patients with HFpEF.[14] Other quality measures, such as blood pressure control and lipid-lowering therapy, were also less commonly met in patients with HFpEF at the time of admission.[15]

PATTERNS OF CARE

Oral agent use during hospitalization and at the time of discharge followed similar patterns to that at the time of initial presentation.[14–16] Uptake of new therapies during admission were low in both cohorts but less pronounced in patients with HFpEF.[14] Approximately 90% of patients were treated during hospitalization with intravenous diuretics, regardless of EF. Although the use of intravenous vasoactive agents was generally low during hospitalization (10%–30%), they were used more frequently in patients with HFrEF.[16] Patients with HFpEF were less likely to undergo any form of procedure, except dialysis, including right-sided and left-sided heart catheterization during hospitalization compared with their HFrEF counterparts.[15]

IN-HOSPITAL MORTALITY

As a continuous variable, similar to studies in ambulatory patients with HF, EF was predictive of in-hospital mortality rates up until an EF of approximately 40%.[14] After this, EF was no longer a significant prognostic indicator of in-hospital mortality. Both the ADHERE and OPTIMIZE-HF showed approximately a 1% absolute increased risk of in-hospital mortality rate in patients with HFrEF compared with HFpEF.[14,16] This finding is consistent with the slightly improved mortality pattern witnessed in patients with outpatient HFpEF compared with HFrEF in a large individual patient data meta-analysis.[18] Rates in the GTWG-HF were more comparable across EF subsets (2.5% in HFpEF vs 2.7% in HFrEF).[15] However, trends over 2005 to 2010 reveal that in-hospital mortality decreased in patients with HFpEF but was stable in patients with HFrEF.[15]

LOS

Average LOS were similar between patients with HFrEF and patients with HFpEF in ADHERE (~5 days)[16] and OPTIMIZE-HF (~6 days).[14] The rate of lengthy hospital stays (>4 days) was more common in patients with HFpEF in unadjusted, but not adjusted, analysis in the GWTG-HF registry.[15] These differences in LOS did not change over time in this registry.[15] LOS seems to be longer in experiences in Europe and Asia, but these international studies are largely limited to HFrEF or mixed EF populations.[19–21]

OTHER IN-HOSPITAL OUTCOMES

Metrics of decongestion including weight loss and change in signs and symptoms of HF during hospitalization were overall similar between clinical subgroups.[14] Patients with HFpEF were more likely to be discharge to skilled nursing or rehabilitation facility compared with patients with HFrEF.[15] Adherence to national performance measures (3 out of 5 of which applies to both EF cohorts) was more common in patients with HFrEF.[14]

POSTDISCHARGE OUTCOMES

EF as a continuous measure is poorly correlated with postdischarge outcomes in the OPTIMIZE-HF registry.[14] This finding is consistent with prior smaller investigations showing that EF is not predictive of recurrent mortality or rehospitalization.[22] Rates of postdischarge mortality and rehospitalization were approximately 10% and 30%, respectively, in both EF-based subgroups at 60 to 90 days of follow-up (**Fig. 2**).[14] Two large population-based studies provide further data

defining the postdischarge clinical course of these two subgroups. In a Canadian experience of 2802 patients admitted with a new HF diagnosis from 1999 to 2001, mortality and readmission rates between HFpEF and HFrEF were similar at 30 days and 1 year.[23] In a 15-year study of 6076 patients with HHF from Olmsted County, patients with HFpEF and patients with HFrEF experienced high rates of mortality at 1 and 5 years. Those patients with HFpEF experienced a slightly better mortality at 1 year (29% vs 32%) and 5 years (65% vs 68%) compared with patients with HFrEF.[24] These small differences persisted after multivariate adjustment. Postdischarge mortality rates improved significantly in HFrEF during the study period but remained unchanged in HFpEF.[24] Based on combined data from large outpatient HFpEF trials, it has been suggested that patients with HFpEF have lower overall hospitalization rates compared with HFrEF in selected populations.[25] In the recent Aliskiren Trial on Acute Heart Failure Outcomes trial, patients with HFrEF in the placebo arm experienced a combined mortality and rehospitalization rate of almost 40% within 6 months of hospital discharge.[26] In high-risk HFrEF subgroups with low systolic blood pressure and renal dysfunction, postdischarge mortality and readmission approach 15% and 30% within 60 to 90 days, respectively.[27]

MODE OF DEATH AND REASONS FOR REHOSPITALIZATION

In patients hospitalized with HFrEF in the trial setting, approximately 40% of postdischarge deaths were secondary to HF alone, whereas 30% were related to sudden cardiac death and

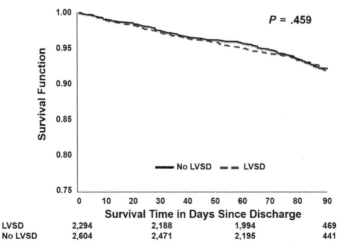

Fig. 2. Survival after hospital discharge. Kaplan-Meier survival curves after hospital discharge in patients with and without LV systolic dysfunction (LVSD) in the follow-up cohort of the Organized Program to Initiate Lifesaving Treatment in Hospitalized Patients with Heart Failure registry. (*Adapted from* Fonarow GC, Stough WG, Abraham WT, et al. Characteristics, treatments, and outcomes of patients with preserved systolic function hospitalized for heart failure: a report from the OPTIMIZE-HF Registry. J Am Coll Cardiol 2007;50(8):768–77; with permission.)

$P = .459$

LVSD	2,294	2,188	1,994	469
No LVSD	2,604	2,471	2,195	441

*P value (40%≤ EF ≤50% vs EF >50%)

another 30% related to noncardiac causes.[28] Similarly, less than half of the patients hospitalized in the postdischarge time frame were hospitalized because of HF alone.[28] Data are presently lacking for mode of death and reasons for rehospitalization in hospitalized patients with HFpEF. Extrapolation from chronic HFpEF trials[29–31] suggests that a larger portion of postdischarge events may be secondary to noncardiac causes in patients with HFpEF.[32]

PREDICTORS OF OUTCOME

In HFpEF and HFrEF, elevated renal parameters (blood urea nitrogen and serum creatinine) and low systolic blood pressure at the time of admission seem to be the strongest in-hospital mortality predictors.[16] Heart rate may have unique predictive ability in patients with HFpEF but not in HFrEF.[16] Similar risk factors and predictors were identified in the subgroup of patients presenting with new-onset HF.[16] The discharge use of beta-blockers, ACE inhibitors, and ARBs was associated with reduced postdischarge mortality and rehospitalization in HFrEF, but not in HFpEF, in propensity-adjusted models in OPTIMIZE-HF.[14] Comprehensive inpatient risk-prediction models are lacking in HFpEF. However, the GWTG-HF risk model for inpatient mortality performed similarly well in both HFpEF and HFrEF in terms of discrimination and calibration (c-index ~0.75).[33] Biomarkers such as natriuretic peptides offered similar risk prediction of in-hospital mortality in the ADHERE registry in HFrEF and HFpEF.[34] In the outpatient setting, an individual patient meta-analysis of almost 40,000 patients in more than 30 chronic HF trials has recently revealed differential risk predictors in HFrEF and HFpEF.[35] Most notably, age was found to be more predictive and systolic blood pressure less predictive of mortality in HFpEF compared with HFrEF.[35]

SUMMARY

HHF represents a population of patients with high postdischarge event rates with relatively limited inpatient targeted therapies. This is particularly true in patients hospitalized with HFpEF. This review characterizes the current clinical landscape of HHF and compares and contrasts HFpEF and HFrEF in terms of baseline characteristics, clinical course, in-hospital and postdischarge outcomes, and predictors of events. The authors have also identified key areas that require further investigation. More standardized EF cut-offs and clinical definitions in HFpEF may be helpful. Limited information is presently available that evaluates

patients with HFpEF in the postdischarge time frame. Risk-prediction models have generally demonstrated similar risk prediction in patients with HFrEF and HFpEF. International experiences are required to corroborate initial registry-based studies in the United States. Finally, evidence-based therapies that can improve outcomes in patients with HFpEF are urgently needed. More complete characterization of this population may be the first step in identifying key areas of potential intervention in hospitalized patients with HFpEF.

REFERENCES

1. Go AS, Mozaffarian D, Roger VL, et al. Executive summary: heart disease and stroke statistics–2013 update: a report from the American Heart Association. Circulation 2013;127(1):143–52.
2. Heidenreich PA, Trogdon JG, Khavjou OA, et al. Forecasting the future of cardiovascular disease in the United States: a policy statement from the American Heart Association. Circulation 2011;123(8): 933–44.
3. Blecker S, Paul M, Taksler G, et al. Heart failure associated hospitalizations in the United States. J Am Coll Cardiol 2013;61(12):1259–67.
4. Chen J, Normand SL, Wang Y, et al. National and regional trends in heart failure hospitalization and mortality rates for Medicare beneficiaries, 1998-2008. JAMA 2011;306(15):1669–78.
5. Jencks SF, Williams MV, Coleman EA. Rehospitalizations among patients in the Medicare fee-for-service program. N Engl J Med 2009;360(14):1418–28.
6. McMurray JJ. Clinical practice. Systolic heart failure. N Engl J Med 2010;362(3):228–38.
7. Gheorghiade M, Vaduganathan M, Fonarow GC, et al. Rehospitalization for heart failure: problems and perspectives. J Am Coll Cardiol 2013;61(4): 391–403.
8. Ahmed A, Allman RM, Fonarow GC, et al. Incident heart failure hospitalization and subsequent mortality in chronic heart failure: a propensity-matched study. J Card Fail 2008;14(3):211–8.
9. Bueno H, Ross JS, Wang Y, et al. Trends in length of stay and short-term outcomes among Medicare patients hospitalized for heart failure, 1993-2006. JAMA 2010;303(21):2141–7.
10. Ross JS, Chen J, Lin Z, et al. Recent national trends in readmission rates after heart failure hospitalization. Circ Heart Fail 2010;3(1):97–103.
11. Chen J, Dharmarajan K, Wang Y, et al. National trends in heart failure hospital stay rates, 2001 to 2009. J Am Coll Cardiol 2013;61(10):1078–88.
12. Caruana L, Petrie MC, Davie AP, et al. Do patients with suspected heart failure and preserved left ventricular systolic function suffer from "diastolic heart

failure" or from misdiagnosis? A prospective descriptive study. BMJ 2000;321(7255):215–8.

13. Paulus WJ, Tschope C, Sanderson JE, et al. How to diagnose diastolic heart failure: a consensus statement on the diagnosis of heart failure with normal left ventricular ejection fraction by the Heart Failure and Echocardiography Associations of the European Society of Cardiology. Eur Heart J 2007; 28(20):2539–50.

14. Fonarow GC, Stough WG, Abraham WT, et al. Characteristics, treatments, and outcomes of patients with preserved systolic function hospitalized for heart failure: a report from the OPTIMIZE-HF Registry. J Am Coll Cardiol 2007;50(8):768–77.

15. Steinberg BA, Zhao X, Heidenreich PA, et al. Trends in patients hospitalized with heart failure and preserved left ventricular ejection fraction: prevalence, therapies, and outcomes. Circulation 2012;126(1): 65–75.

16. Yancy CW, Lopatin M, Stevenson LW, et al. Clinical presentation, management, and in-hospital outcomes of patients admitted with acute decompensated heart failure with preserved systolic function: a report from the Acute Decompensated Heart Failure National Registry (ADHERE) database. J Am Coll Cardiol 2006;47(1):76–84.

17. Brouwers FP, de Boer RA, van der Harst P, et al. Incidence and epidemiology of new onset heart failure with preserved vs. reduced ejection fraction in a community-based cohort: 11-year follow-up of PRE-VEND. Eur Heart J, in press.

18. Meta-analysis Global Group in Chronic Heart Failure. The survival of patients with heart failure with preserved or reduced left ventricular ejection fraction: an individual patient data meta-analysis. Eur Heart J 2012;33(14):1750–7.

19. Chioncel O, Vinereanu D, Datcu M, et al. The Romanian Acute Heart Failure Syndromes (RO-AHFS) registry. Am Heart J 2011;162(1):142–153.e1.

20. Sato N, Kajimoto K, Asai K, et al. Acute decompensated heart failure syndromes (ATTEND) registry. A prospective observational multicenter cohort study: rationale, design, and preliminary data. Am Heart J 2010;159(6):949–955.e1.

21. Tavazzi L, Maggioni AP, Lucci D, et al. Nationwide survey on acute heart failure in cardiology ward services in Italy. Eur Heart J 2006;27(10):1207–15.

22. Solomon SD, Dobson J, Pocock S, et al. Influence of nonfatal hospitalization for heart failure on subsequent mortality in patients with chronic heart failure. Circulation 2007;116(13):1482–7.

23. Bhatia RS, Tu JV, Lee DS, et al. Outcome of heart failure with preserved ejection fraction in a population-based study. N Engl J Med 2006; 355(3):260–9.

24. Owan TE, Hodge DO, Herges RM, et al. Trends in prevalence and outcome of heart failure with preserved ejection fraction. N Engl J Med 2006; 355(3):251–9.

25. Campbell RT, Jhund PS, Castagno D, et al. What have we learned about patients with heart failure and preserved ejection fraction from DIG-PEF, CHARM-preserved, and I-PRESERVE? J Am Coll Cardiol 2012;60(23):2349–56.

26. Gheorghiade M, Bohm M, Greene SJ, et al. Effect of aliskiren on postdischarge mortality and heart failure readmissions among patients hospitalized for heart failure: the ASTRONAUT randomized trial. JAMA 2013;309(11):1125–35.

27. Gheorghiade M, Abraham WT, Albert NM, et al. Systolic blood pressure at admission, clinical characteristics, and outcomes in patients hospitalized with acute heart failure. JAMA 2006;296(18): 2217–26.

28. O'Connor CM, Miller AB, Blair JE, et al. Causes of death and rehospitalization in patients hospitalized with worsening heart failure and reduced left ventricular ejection fraction: results from Efficacy of Vasopressin Antagonism in Heart Failure Outcome Study with Tolvaptan (EVEREST) program. Am Heart J 2010;159(5):841–849.e1.

29. Ahmed A, Rich MW, Fleg JL, et al. Effects of digoxin on morbidity and mortality in diastolic heart failure: the Ancillary Digitalis Investigation Group trial. Circulation 2006;114(5):397–403.

30. Yusuf S, Pfeffer MA, Swedberg K, et al. Effects of candesartan in patients with chronic heart failure and preserved left-ventricular ejection fraction: the CHARM-Preserved Trial. Lancet 2003;362(9386): 777–81.

31. Zile MR, Gaasch WH, Anand IS, et al. Mode of death in patients with heart failure and a preserved ejection fraction: results from the Irbesartan in Heart Failure With Preserved Ejection Fraction Study (I-Preserve) trial. Circulation 2010;121(12):1393–405.

32. Shah SJ, Gheorghiade M. Heart failure with preserved ejection fraction: treat now by treating comorbidities. JAMA 2008;300(4):431–3.

33. Peterson PN, Rumsfeld JS, Liang L, et al. A validated risk score for in-hospital mortality in patients with heart failure from the American Heart Association get with the guidelines program. Circ Cardiovasc Qual Outcomes 2010;3(1):25–32.

34. Fonarow GC, Peacock WF, Phillips CO, et al. Admission B-type natriuretic peptide levels and in-hospital mortality in acute decompensated heart failure. J Am Coll Cardiol 2007;49(19):1943–50.

35. Pocock SJ, Ariti CA, McMurray JJ, et al. Predicting survival in heart failure: a risk score based on 39 372 patients from 30 studies. Eur Heart J, in press.

Classification of Patients Hospitalized for Heart Failure

Muthiah Vaduganathan, MD, MPH[a],
Catherine N. Marti, MD[b], Vasiliki V. Georgiopoulou, MD[b],
Andreas P. Kalogeropoulos, MD, PhD[b],
Javed Butler, MD, MPH[b],*

KEYWORDS

- Acute heart failure • Classification • Management • Outcomes

KEY POINTS

- Approximately 90% of patients hospitalized with heart failure (HHF) are managed with intravenous diuretics and few patients are initiated on new therapies during admission.
- Many HHF patients have 1 or more clearly identifiable precipitants driving the requirement for hospitalization.
- Social determinants of health, such as access to care, income, and mental illness, have a major influence on hospitalization and postdischarge outcomes in HHF.
- Approximately 15% to 20% of HHF patients present with new-onset or newly diagnosed HF and less than 5% have end-stage HF.
- HHF is not a single disease but represents the endpoint for several cardiac and noncardiac processes.

INTRODUCTION

Heart failure (HF) affects more than 5 million patients every year and is the leading cause of hospitalizations and rehospitalizations among older adults in the United States.[1] HF prevalence and incidence are poised to rise in upcoming years based on the aging demographic.[2] Patients hospitalized for HF (HHF) experience significant symptomatic improvement with standard diuretic regimens[3] and are at low risk of in-hospital mortality, regardless of ejection fraction (EF).[4–6] Recent studies reveal improvements in various quality metrics, including length of stay and in-hospital mortality.[7] Despite these, HHF patients experience rates of postdischarge mortality and rehospitalization approaching 15% and 30% within 60 to 90 days over the last decade.[8] Even in well-treated, well-monitored populations in large, recent randomized controlled trials, combined event rates are approximately 40% within 6 months of hospital discharge.[9] These morbidity and mortality figures are similar to those of many cancers and higher than those reported in acute myocardial infarction.[10] Total HF-related admissions[11] and readmissions[12] have been unwaveringly steady over the past several years.

Heterogeneity Among HHF Patients

Despite advancements in the overall HF drug and device armamentarium for patients with chronic HF with low EF,[13] management of HHF patients remains inadequate. A major challenge facing

Disclosures: No relevant relationships to disclose for all authors.
[a] Department of Medicine, Massachusetts General Hospital, Harvard Medical School, 55 Fruit Street, GRB 740, Boston, MA 02114, USA; [b] Division of Cardiology, Emory University School of Medicine, Emory Clinical Cardiovascular Research Institute, 1462 Clifton Road Northeast, Suite 504, Atlanta, GA 30322, USA
* Corresponding author.
E-mail address: javed.butler@emory.edu

heartfailure.theclinics.com

clinicians and researchers is the marked heterogeneity in clinical profiles within HHF patients.[14] From initial presentation in the emergency department to postdischarge clinical courses, HHF patients differ in terms of their clinical characteristics, prognostic markers, precipitating factors, and cardiac and noncardiac comorbidities. Even region-based and site-based differences have been recently identified in selected global HF populations.[15,16] These parameters each uniquely inform management practices. Poor patient selection may be a major contributing reason for recent trial failure.[17] Improved classification schemes for HHF may assist in both clinical and research settings to match individual patients with tailored management approaches.

Classification Dilemma

Traditional classification schemes using the American College of Cardiology/American Heart Association (ACC/AHA) staging and New York Heart Association functional classes have been used for decades in the outpatient setting. They may have poor applicability, however, in patients with rapidly changing hemodynamic and clinical status who are hospitalized with HF. Gheorghiade and Braunwald[18] proposed an initial model for the assessment of HHF patients at first presentation. This 6-axis model uses readily available clinical information including vital signs to rapidly risk-stratify patients. The model incorporates clinical severity, blood pressure, heart rate, and rhythm, precipitants, comorbidities, and de novo versus chronic HF.[18] The model may be useful primarily for initial triage and immediate clinical care at the time of admission. Limited risk-stratification models during hospitalization exist to guide further management and disposition. Many proposed models, however, are largely outcomes focused and do not directly inform clinical decision making. Several of these models require data on several parameters that may not be readily available for all HHF patients.[19] Furthermore, many contemporary classification schemes do not address patients with HF and preserved EF (HFpEF). The American Heart Association Get With The Guidelines–Heart Failure (GWTG-HF) inpatient mortality model seems to have similar prognostic value in patients with preserved EF and reduced EF, however.[20] This article proposes a practical, management-based approach to classification of HHF patients.

PROPOSED CLASSIFICATION SCHEME

Several clinically important variables likely influence endpoints after discharge in HF, but few may be modifiable and uniquely targeted with available therapies. Although data in this area continue to evolve, this article identifies key parameters that may help inform clinicians regarding strategies of inpatient and postdischarge management. This classification scheme (**Fig. 1**) divides patients sequentially based on the following variables: (1) EF, (2) medical or social precipitants, and (3) chronicity of HF.

Ejection Fraction

Based on its original nomenclature, *heart failure* has carried the connotation that the heart is

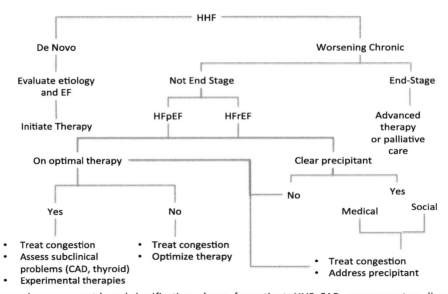

Fig. 1. Proposed management-based classification scheme for patients HHF. CAD, coronary artery disease.

unable to pump, thereby implying a low EF. It is now widely acknowledged, however, that a large proportion of patients with HF have HFpEF. Originally thought simply a precursor to HF with reduced EF (HFrEF), this clinical entity is distinguished by unique epidemiology, clinical profiles, prognostic markers, therapeutic targets, and management approaches. The widespread availability of contemporary imaging techniques and biomarkers has provided key tools to better characterize HFpEF. A consensus statement[21] from the Heart Failure Association and Echocardiography Association of the European Society of Cardiology has helped establish clear diagnostic criteria for this syndrome. The diagnosis requires (1) the presence of signs and symptoms of congestion, (2) normal or near-normal systolic function, and (3) evidence of diastolic dysfunction.[21] Approximately 50% to 55% of all HF patients have HFpEF based in both inpatient[4–6] and outpatient[22] care settings. The overall prevalence of HFpEF is 1.1% to 5.5% in these community-based investigations but increases with age and in women.[22] HFpEF patients are more likely to be female and older and to have a history of hypertension and are less likely to have ischemic HF etiology.[4–6] Despite slightly improved inpatient mortality patterns, HFpEF patients face similar postdischarge outcomes as patients with HFrEF.[23,24] The majority of current national guideline recommendations for the management of HF apply almost exclusively to patients with HFrEF.[13] Clinical trials in HFpEF have yet to be completed; thus, the management approach in these patients remains empiric. Due to the high burden of comorbid illness and non–cardiovascular-related postdischarge events, stringent risk factor modification in this population is recommended.[25]

Medical Precipitants

Data from the Organized Program to Initiate Lifesaving Treatment in Hospitalized Patients with Heart Failure (OPTIMIZE-HF) registry represents the most comprehensive description of precipitants and reasons for initial presentation in HHF patients.[26] Of the approximately 50,000 patients included in the study, roughly 60% had 1 or more clearly identified precipitating factor. Medical precipitants of HHF can be broadly categorized as cardiac and noncardiac. Cardiac precipitants most commonly include myocardial ischemia[27]; arrhythmias, especially atrial fibrillation[28]; and uncontrolled hypertension.[29] The relative contribution of heart rate and blood pressure may be more pronounced in patients with HFpEF.[4] Noncardiac causes most commonly involve pneumonia and worsening renal function. The roles of chronic obstructive pulmonary disease,[30] diabetes,[31] and obstructive sleep apnea, however, are becoming increasingly recognized in HHF outcomes. A high index of clinical suspicion for these factors should be maintained to help identify these precipitants at an early stage during hospitalization. The OPTIMIZE-HF data revealed that these precipitants independently predict clinical outcomes; thus, tailored therapies addressing these triggering mechanisms should be promptly and thoroughly instituted.

Other Precipitants

Patients without a clear medical trigger to their current HF hospitalization (approximately 40%) may have a definite social cause underlying their exacerbation. These factors include medication noncompliance, dietary indiscretions, and drug and alcohol use/abuse. Targeted interventions improving compliance patterns may help ameliorate outcomes in HF.[32] Multidisciplinary teams, including physicians, nurses, pharmacists, dieticians, and social workers, may help improve overall care and patient outcomes.[33,34] The postdischarge period represents a dynamic and difficult transition for patients to their home environment (**Box 1**). National efforts, such as the ACC Hospital to Home initiative[35] and the AHA GWTG-HF and Target: HF programs,[36] are aimed at easing the inpatient to outpatient transition. Telemonitoring does not seem to have a central role in care transition and postdischarge follow-up of patients recently hospitalized for HF.[37] Joynt and Jha[38] highlight the important social and racial determinants for readmission risk in HHF. Factors, such as mental illness, social support, and socioeconomic status, may be difficult to modify even with targeted approaches.

De Novo Heart Failure

HHF patients can be divided into patients with de novo (approximately 15%–20%) or worsening chronic HF (approximately 80%).[39] Few data are available exploring the epidemiology and clinical course of patients presenting with new HF, given that this subset is largely excluded from major clinical trials. Recent data from the Prevention of Renal and Vascular End-stage Disease study[40] and the Cardiovascular Health Study[41] have begun to define the clinical profile of this important subgroup. A thorough assessment of cardiac function (to document baseline EF), etiology (including an ischemic evaluation), initiating mechanisms, and amplifying factors should be pursued in these patients.

Box 1
List of potential breakdowns in transitions of care for heart failure

Typical breakdowns associated with patient assessment

Failure to actively include the patient and family caregivers in identifying needs, resources, and planning for the discharge

Failure to recognize worsening clinical status before discharge from the hospital

Failure to identify or address comorbid conditions (underlying depression, anemia, hypothyroidism, and so forth)

Medication errors and adverse drug events caused by patient or family-caregiver confusion

Typical breakdowns found in and family caregiver education

Failure to clarify if patient and caregiver understood instructions and plan of care

Failure to address prior nonadherence in self-care, diet, medications, therapies, daily weights, follow-up, and testing

Providing information on broad themes without details on how to make it work for individual patients based on lifestyle, economic constraints, social support, and other patient or process factors

Typical breakdowns in handoff communication

Lack of communication resulting in primary care provider not knowing patients admitted

Poor communication of the care plan to the nursing home team, home health care team, primary care physician, or family caregiver

Discharge instructions missing, inadequate, incomplete, or illegible

Lack of understanding by the health care receiver of information regarding HF medical and self-care management

Typical breakdowns after discharge from the hospital

Medication errors

Patient lack of adherence to self-care (eg, medications, therapies, diet [sodium restriction], and/or daily weights) because of poor understanding or confusion about needed care, how to get appointments, or how to access or pay for medications

No follow-up appointment or follow-up too long after hospitalization

Failure to provide phone number of physician/nurse patient should call if HF worsens

Adapted from Gheorghiade M, Vaduganathan M, Fonarow GC, et al. Rehospitalization for heart failure: problems and perspectives. J Am Coll Cardiol 2013;61:391–403; with permission.

End-Stage Heart Failure

A small percentage (<5%) of HHF patients are end stage[39] and may not respond to standard inpatient therapies. These patients may have low cardiac output and low systemic blood pressure, significantly limiting ability to initiate and up-titrate major life-prolonging therapies.[42] Thus, inotropes and other vasoactive agents are often required in their inpatient management,[5,43] despite their known adverse effects on long-term outcomes.[42] Replacement of the viable myocardium with scar tissue may prevent adequate recovery of ventricular function in this population. The search for a safe inotrope continues that can effectively improve cardiac output and systemic perfusion without concomitant adverse effects on heart rate, myocardial oxygen consumption, renal function, and mortality. More realistically, these patients may benefit from more definite measures, including left ventricular assist device placement or cardiac transplantation. Despite their increased risk of death, few patients with end-stage HF use palliative care services and hospice care.[44] Appropriate and early referral of these patients may improve quality of life outcomes in this population.

Worsening Chronic Heart Failure

A subset of patients with HF is hospitalized despite having been optimized on evidence-based therapies, which may represent therapeutic inadequacy and identify patients amenable for further therapies. Unfortunately, large inpatient registries suggest that the majority of HHF patients are treated the same. Approximately 90% of patients are treated with intravenous diuretics and initiation of new therapies during hospitalization remains low.[5,43] Furthermore, a majority of large phase III clinical trials conducted in HHF have been neutral or negative.[17] A significant number of patients are discharged from the hospital with clinical signs and symptoms of persistent congestion.[3] Adequate decongestion during hospitalization remains the mainstay of HHF management. Endpoints for diuresis are poorly defined and represent an area of active clinical research. Future clinical studies in this population should help to (1) define intensity, duration, and optimal type of fluid removal strategy and (2) find new effective therapies that influence postdischarge outcomes.

SUMMARY

HHF represents a widely heterogeneous population with distinct clinical subsets requiring tailored management approaches. The assessment of EF, precipitants, and chronicity of HF may help stratify patients early during hospitalization to guide subsequent therapeutic strategies. Future work should be aimed at standardizing and validating these schemes in large, prospectively defined populations. A 1-size-fits-all approach to HHF is antiquated. Clinicians and researchers alike should actively identify individual clinical phenotypes to focus management efforts. HHF is not a single disease but a manifestation of several cardiac and noncardiac processes and thus should be approached as such.

REFERENCES

1. Go AS, Mozaffarian D, Roger VL, et al. Executive summary: heart disease and stroke statistics—2013 update: a report from the American Heart Association. Circulation 2013;127:143–52.
2. Heidenreich PA, Trogdon JG, Khavjou OA, et al. Forecasting the future of cardiovascular disease in the United States: a policy statement from the American Heart Association. Circulation 2011;123:933–44.
3. Ambrosy AP, Pang PS, Khan S, et al. Clinical course and predictive value of congestion during hospitalization in patients admitted for worsening signs and symptoms of heart failure with reduced ejection fraction: findings from the EVEREST trial. Eur Heart J 2013;34:835–43.
4. Yancy CW, Lopatin M, Stevenson LW, et al. Clinical presentation, management, and in-hospital outcomes of patients admitted with acute decompensated heart failure with preserved systolic function: a report from the Acute Decompensated Heart Failure National Registry (ADHERE) Database. J Am Coll Cardiol 2006;47:76–84.
5. Fonarow GC, Stough WG, Abraham WT, et al. Characteristics, treatments, and outcomes of patients with preserved systolic function hospitalized for heart failure: a report from the OPTIMIZE-HF Registry. J Am Coll Cardiol 2007;50:768–77.
6. Steinberg BA, Zhao X, Heidenreich PA, et al. Trends in patients hospitalized with heart failure and preserved left ventricular ejection fraction: prevalence, therapies, and outcomes. Circulation 2012;126:65–75.
7. Bueno H, Ross JS, Wang Y, et al. Trends in length of stay and short-term outcomes among Medicare patients hospitalized for heart failure, 1993-2006. JAMA 2010;303:2141–7.
8. Gheorghiade M, Abraham WT, Albert NM, et al. Systolic blood pressure at admission, clinical characteristics, and outcomes in patients hospitalized with acute heart failure. JAMA 2006;296:2217–26.
9. Gheorghiade M, Bohm M, Greene SJ, et al. Effect of aliskiren on postdischarge mortality and heart failure readmissions among patients hospitalized for heart failure: the ASTRONAUT randomized trial. JAMA 2013;309:1125–35.
10. Kostis WJ, Deng Y, Pantazopoulos JS, et al. Myocardial Infarction Data Acquisition System Study G. Trends in mortality of acute myocardial infarction after discharge from the hospital. Circ Cardiovasc Qual Outcomes 2010;3:581–9.
11. Blecker S, Paul M, Taksler G, et al. Heart failure associated hospitalizations in the United States. J Am Coll Cardiol 2013;61:1259–67.
12. Ross JS, Chen J, Lin Z, et al. Recent national trends in readmission rates after heart failure hospitalization. Circ Heart Fail 2010;3:97–103.
13. Jessup M, Abraham WT, Casey DE, et al. 2009 focused update: ACCF/AHA Guidelines for the Diagnosis and Management of Heart Failure in Adults: a report of the American College of Cardiology Foundation/American Heart Association Task Force on Practice Guidelines: developed in collaboration with the International Society for Heart and Lung Transplantation. Circulation 2009;119:1977–2016.
14. Gheorghiade M, Vaduganathan M, Fonarow GC, et al. Rehospitalization for heart failure: problems and perspectives. J Am Coll Cardiol 2013;61:391–403.
15. Blair JE, Zannad F, Konstam MA, et al. Continental differences in clinical characteristics, management, and outcomes in patients hospitalized with worsening heart failure results from the EVEREST (Efficacy of Vasopressin Antagonism in Heart Failure: Outcome Study with Tolvaptan) program. J Am Coll Cardiol 2008;52:1640–8.

16. Butler J, Subacius H, Vaduganathan M, et al. Relationship between clinical trial site enrollment with participant characteristics, protocol completion, and outcomes: insights from the EVEREST (Efficacy of Vasopressin Antagonism in Heart Failure: Outcome Study with Tolvaptan) trial. J Am Coll Cardiol 2013;61:571–9.

17. Vaduganathan M, Greene SJ, Ambrosy AP, et al. The disconnect between phase II and phase III trials of drugs for heart failure. Nat Rev Cardiol 2013;10: 85–97.

18. Gheorghiade M, Braunwald E. A proposed model for initial assessment and management of acute heart failure syndromes. JAMA 2011;305:1702–3.

19. Fonarow GC, Adams KF Jr, Abraham WT, et al. Risk stratification for in-hospital mortality in acutely decompensated heart failure: classification and regression tree analysis. JAMA 2005;293:572–80.

20. Peterson PN, Rumsfeld JS, Liang L, et al. A validated risk score for in-hospital mortality in patients with heart failure from the American Heart Association get with the guidelines program. Circ Cardiovasc Qual Outcomes 2010;3:25–32.

21. Paulus WJ, Tschope C, Sanderson JE, et al. How to diagnose diastolic heart failure: a consensus statement on the diagnosis of heart failure with normal left ventricular ejection fraction by the Heart Failure and Echocardiography Associations of the European Society of Cardiology. Eur Heart J 2007;28: 2539–50.

22. Owan TE, Redfield MM. Epidemiology of diastolic heart failure. Prog Cardiovasc Dis 2005;47:320–32.

23. Bhatia RS, Tu JV, Lee DS, et al. Outcome of heart failure with preserved ejection fraction in a population-based study. N Engl J Med 2006;355: 260–9.

24. Owan TE, Hodge DO, Herges RM, et al. Trends in prevalence and outcome of heart failure with preserved ejection fraction. N Engl J Med 2006;355: 251–9.

25. Shah SJ, Gheorghiade M. Heart failure with preserved ejection fraction: treat now by treating comorbidities. JAMA 2008;300:431–3.

26. Fonarow GC, Abraham WT, Albert NM, et al. Factors identified as precipitating hospital admissions for heart failure and clinical outcomes: findings from OPTIMIZE-HF. Arch Intern Med 2008;168:847–54.

27. Mentz RJ, Allen BD, Kwasny MJ, et al. Influence of documented history of coronary artery disease on outcomes in patients admitted for worsening heart failure with reduced ejection fraction in the EVEREST trial. Eur J Heart Fail 2013;15:61–8.

28. Mentz RJ, Chung MJ, Gheorghiade M, et al. Atrial fibrillation or flutter on initial electrocardiogram is associated with worse outcomes in patients admitted for worsening heart failure with reduced ejection fraction: findings from the EVEREST Trial. Am Heart J 2012;164:884–892.e2.

29. Ambrosy AP, Vaduganathan M, Mentz RJ, et al. Clinical profile and prognostic value of low systolic blood pressure in patients hospitalized for heart failure with reduced ejection fraction: insights from the Efficacy of Vasopressin Antagonism in Heart Failure: Outcome Study with Tolvaptan (EVEREST) trial. Am Heart J 2013;165:216–25.

30. Mentz RJ, Schmidt PH, Kwasny MJ, et al. The impact of chronic obstructive pulmonary disease in patients hospitalized for worsening heart failure with reduced ejection fraction: an analysis of the EVEREST Trial. J Card Fail 2012;18:515–23.

31. Sarma S, Mentz RJ, Kwasny MJ, et al. Association between diabetes mellitus and post-discharge outcomes in patients hospitalized with heart failure: findings from the EVEREST trial. Eur J Heart Fail 2013;15:194–202.

32. McAlister FA, Lawson FM, Teo KK, et al. A systematic review of randomized trials of disease management programs in heart failure. Am J Med 2001;110:378–84.

33. Holland R, Battersby J, Harvey I, et al. Systematic review of multidisciplinary interventions in heart failure. Heart 2005;91:899–906.

34. McAlister FA, Stewart S, Ferrua S, et al. Multidisciplinary strategies for the management of heart failure patients at high risk for admission: a systematic review of randomized trials. J Am Coll Cardiol 2004;44:810–9.

35. Wiggins BS, Rodgers JE, Didomenico RJ, et al. Discharge counseling for patients with heart failure or myocardial infarction: a best practices model developed by Members of the American College of Clinical Pharmacy's Cardiology Practice and Research Network Based on the Hospital to Home (H2H) Initiative. Pharmacotherapy 2013;33: 558–80.

36. Heidenreich PA, Hernandez AF, Yancy CW, et al. Get with the guidelines program participation, process of care, and outcome for Medicare patients hospitalized with heart failure. Circ Cardiovasc Qual Outcomes 2012;5:37–43.

37. Chaudhry SI, Mattera JA, Curtis JP, et al. Telemonitoring in patients with heart failure. N Engl J Med 2010;363:2301–9.

38. Joynt KE, Jha AK. Thirty-day readmissions—truth and consequences. N Engl J Med 2012;366:1366–9.

39. Gheorghiade M, Pang PS. Acute heart failure syndromes. J Am Coll Cardiol 2009;53:557–73.

40. Brouwers FP, de Boer RA, van der Harst P, et al. Incidence and epidemiology of new onset heart failure with preserved vs. reduced ejection fraction in a community-based cohort: 11-year follow-up of PREVEND. Eur Heart J 2013. [Epub ahead of print].

41. Chaudhry SI, McAvay G, Chen S, et al. Risk factors for hospital admission among older persons with newly diagnosed heart failure: findings from the Cardiovascular Health Study. J Am Coll Cardiol 2013; 61:635–42.

42. Gheorghiade M, Vaduganathan M, Ambrosy A, et al. Current management and future directions for the treatment of patients hospitalized for heart failure with low blood pressure. Heart Fail Rev 2013;18: 107–22.

43. Adams KF Jr, Fonarow GC, Emerman CL, et al. Characteristics and outcomes of patients hospitalized for heart failure in the United States: rationale, design, and preliminary observations from the first 100,000 cases in the Acute Decompensated Heart Failure National Registry (ADHERE). Am Heart J 2005;149:209–16.

44. Whellan DJ, Cox M, Hernandez AF, et al. Utilization of hospice and predicted mortality risk among older patients hospitalized with heart failure: findings from GWTG-HF. J Card Fail 2012;18:471–7.

Recognizing Hospitalized Heart Failure as an Entity and Developing New Therapies to Improve Outcomes
Academics', Clinicians', Industry's, Regulators', and Payers' Perspectives

Mihai Gheorghiade, MD[a],*, Ami N. Shah, MD[a],
Muthiah Vaduganathan, MD, MPH[b], Javed Butler, MD, MPH[c],
Robert O. Bonow, MD, MS[a], Giuseppe M.C. Rosano, MD, PhD[d],
Scott Taylor, RPh, MBA[e], Stuart Kupfer, MD[f], Frank Misselwitz, MD, PhD[g],
Arjun Sharma, MD[h], Gregg C. Fonarow, MD[i]

KEYWORDS

• Hospitalized heart failure • Heart failure • Postdischarge mortality

KEY POINTS

• Hospitalized heart failure (HHF) is associated with unacceptably high postdischarge mortality and rehospitalization rates.
• This heterogeneous group of patients, however, is still treated with standard, homogenous therapies that are not preventing their rapid deterioration.
• The costs associated with HHF have added demands from society, government, and payers to improve outcomes.
• It is important to consider that once HHF patients are stabilized by discharge, the majority of them should be considered to be in a chronic heart failure state at a significantly high risk for adverse outcomes. Delaying initiation of potentially effective therapies for weeks to months post discharge risks unabated high risk for adverse events in the meantime. Initiating therapies in patients who are stabilized in the hospital and continued long term provides a potent option to improve long-term clinical outcomes.
• With coordinated and committed efforts in the development of new therapies, improvements may be seen in outcomes for patients with HHF.
• This article summarizes concepts in developing therapies for HHF discussed during a multidisciplinary panel at the Heart Failure Society of America's Annual Scientific Meeting, September 2012.

Disclosures: See last page of article.
[a] Center for Cardiovascular Innovation, Northwestern University Feinberg School of Medicine, 645 North Michigan Avenue, Chicago, IL 60611, USA; [b] Department of Medicine, Massachusetts General Hospital, Harvard Medical School, 55 Fruit Street, Boston, MA 02114, USA; [c] Division of Cardiology, Emory University School of Medicine, 1364 Clifton Road, Atlanta, GA 30322, USA; [d] Division of Cardiology, IRCC San Raffaele, 235 Via della Pisana 00163, Rome, Italy; [e] Industry Relations, Geisinger Health System, 100 N Academy Avenue, Danville, PA 17822, USA; [f] Takeda Global Research and Development Center, Inc., 1 Takeda Parkway, Deerfield, IL 60015, USA; [g] Bayer HealthCare Pharmaceuticals, 178 Müllerstr 13353, Berlin, Germany; [h] Ontario Ministry of Health and Long-Term Care, 80 Grosvenor Street, Ontario, Canada; [i] Division of Cardiology, UCLA, 10833 LeConte Avenue, Los Angeles, CA 90024, USA
* Corresponding author. Center for Cardiovascular Innovation, Northwestern University Feinberg School of Medicine, 645 North Michigan Avenue, Suite 1006, Chicago, IL 60611.
E-mail address: m-gheorghiade@northwestern.edu

Heart Failure Clin 9 (2013) 285–290
http://dx.doi.org/10.1016/j.hfc.2013.05.002
1551-7136/13/$ – see front matter © 2013 Published by Elsevier Inc.

INTRODUCTION

HF is a syndrome with common clinical manifestations of diverse cardiac and noncardiac abnormalities. These differences have implications for outcomes and for development of new therapies; therefore, it is necessary to define and classify HF patients appropriately. A broad classification is to divide patients into outpatients and those with HHF and, secondarily, those with reduced versus preserved ejection fraction. These distinctions are important because they represent groups with different underlying pathophysiologic, hemodynamic, and neurohormonal abnormalities and with varying outcomes and responses to existing therapies.

HOSPITALIZED HEART FAILURE: AN IMPORTANT DISTINCT ENTITY

HF is present in more than 6.6 million Americans with a 5-year survival ranging from 26% to 52% in studies where incident HF was adjudicated as first HHF for participants.[1,2] The prevalence of HF is expected to increase 25% by 2030.[2] HF is the primary cause of 1 million admissions and the secondary cause of another 2 million hospitalizations annually.[3] Although mortality for outpatients has decreased and remains low, the mortality for patients with HHF is approximately 15% at 60 to 90 days and reaches 30% a 1 year.[2,4–6] One in 4 patients with HHF is readmitted within 30 days.[7] Recurrent admissions for HHF are associated with worsening of chronic HF and higher mortality.[8] Nevertheless, aside from the small portion of patients with HHF who have end-stage disease, most have the potential for recovery.[9] Since 2009 the Centers for Medicare and Medicaid Services have been publicly reporting 30-day rehospitalization rates for HF, and now readmission rates among HHF patients have begun to affect Medicare reimbursement.[10,11]

Given the high mortality, morbidity, and costs associated with HHF, there is an enormous unmet need for drugs and devices that improve outcomes for these patients.

Despite several large clinical trials with the participation of thousands of patients and an incredible resource investment, no new therapies have emerged for improving HHF outcomes. There are several reasons for this; chief among them is lack of recognition of HHF as an entity.[12] HHF trials have mostly focused on improving transient short-term symptoms with a 1- to 2-day intervention, whereas long-term interventions have largely been tested on stable outpatients. It is imperative to recognize that the problem with HHF is not in-hospital but postdischarge outcomes. Therefore, the major problem with HHF has neither been addressed by acute HF trials focused on short-term symptoms nor by chronic HF trials targeting stable outpatients.

HHF as an entity identifying a high-risk group for adverse outcomes postdischarge is important for the patient population, researchers, clinicians, industry, payers, and regulators alike. Targeting postdischarge outcomes in HHF patients represents one of the most urgent unmet needs in medicine.

DEVELOPING THERAPIES FOR HOSPITALIZED HEART FAILURE PATIENTS

Development of drugs and devices for HHF requires deliberate efforts to improve study design and execution in the setting of heightened cooperation and communication among all stakeholders. Several key elements in developing HHF therapies are discussed.

Knowing the Drug or Device

It is important to thoroughly understanding the drug or device studied in order to develop effective trials. Phase III trials have been often conducted with limited knowledge of a drug's mechanism of action, impact on cardiovascular and noncardiovascular parameters, toxicities, and dosing[13,14]; hence, most of the promising results from phase II studies have not translated to benefit in phase III. Success with phase III trials might occur if they are designed after a thorough mechanistic understanding of a drug and its effects on the pathophysiologic state being explored. A T1 phase trial may help bridge animal data with phase II trials[13] by conducting trials in a small, homogenous population (eg, a narrow age range, ejection fraction, background therapy, and renal function) for hypothesis testing. With more thorough early investigations, the ideal target substrate or patient population can be defined along with expected safety concerns. T1 testing can also help define the dose, timing, frequency, and duration of treatment that achieves most benefit but avoids toxicities.

Matching Intervention with the Patient

Given the HHF phenotypic diversity, therapies that do not benefit or that harm large unselected patients may benefit particular subgroups. It is important to conduct investigations in patients with the phenotype and pathophysiology most likely to benefit. For example, rolofylline, an A1 adenosine receptor antagonist, was expected to affect the downstream effects of afferent vasoconstriction and sodium reabsorption.[15–17] A phase III trial tested the hypothesis that HHF patients are at a high risk for worsening renal function and that rolofylline preserves renal function, translating into improved outcomes; however, in more than 2000 patients, there was no difference in clinical outcomes.[18] The efficacy of the drug, however, may not have been adequately tested because less than 10% of enrolled patients developed worsening renal function in this study.[19] To match the therapy with the right patients, many factors must be considered, based on cause, ejection fraction, signs and symptoms, blood pressure and rhythm, comorbidities, background therapies, hemodynamic profile, renal function, and volume of distribution. Biomarkers or other studies (eg, viability studies) may help identify a subgroup that may have greatest benefit. The benefits and risks may be realized at different times (eg, devices have high upfront risks but the benefits are realized later).[20] Thus, patients selected for device trials should have an expected life expectancy to realize the benefit.

Meaningful Endpoints

Trials achieve clinically significant improvement within a reassuring safety profile. Traditionally, regulatory agencies have required endpoints indicating improved life expectancy or symptoms, because drugs improving surrogate endpoints have failed to show a survival benefit or have a detrimental effect. Although dyspnea is often targeted as an endpoint, diuretics improve dyspnea within a few hours[21–23] and dyspnea lacks correlation with long-term outcomes.[24–27] With the efficacy of current therapies, new therapies targeting dyspnea typically require large trials to demonstrate incremental benefit. Given the variability in dyspnea measurement, it is important to have objective evidence of effectiveness. Therefore, early improvement in dyspnea may be considered as an endpoint only if supported by improved congestion or reduction in pulmonary wedge pressure. In the absence of a compelling benefit in mortality or clinically meaningful morbidity, a significant amount of reassuring safety data are needed to justify the likely small incremental acute improvement of dyspnea.[28] With the low cost and high efficacy of current therapies, a small improvement in dyspnea would likely not meet payer demands for cost-effective improvement in outcomes. Thus, instead of focusing on short-term dyspnea relief, new therapies should benefit meaningful outcomes, such as mortality, hospitalization, and long-term functional status.

Timing and Duration of Interventions

Standard therapies for HHF improve symptoms but do not curb the mortality and hospitalization rates after discharge. Most interventions in HHF trials were initiated in the first 24 to 48 hours of HHF and continued for a few days during the inpatient stay, making it unlikely to demonstrate improvements in outcomes weeks to months later.[29–34] Therefore it is important to consider that once HHF patients are stabilized by the time of discharge, the majority of them should be considered to be in a chronic heart failure state but at a significantly higher risk for adverse outcomes. Delaying initiation of potentially effective therapies for weeks to months post discharge risks unabated high risk for adverse events in the meantime. Initiating therapies in HHF patients who are stabilized in the hospital and continued long term provides a potent option to improve long-term clinical outcomes among these patients.

Beyond Megatrials

Phase III trials in HHF have tested potential therapies on a broad spectrum of hundreds to thousands of heterogeneous patients with neutral or deleterious effects. Most HHF patients are already on multiple medications and the layering on of additional drugs in a one-size-fits-all manner has been ineffective. The large number of patients in current trials contributes to mounting costs and a lengthy enrollment period. Yet megatrials may be unnecessary given the high event rate postdischarge. With effective therapy, a statically and clinically meaningful improvement in outcomes should be discernible in smaller populations. Changing the focus from megatrials to a more personalized approach with new therapies may have a higher yield. For example, a therapy targeted for 20% of HHF patients that offered 20% improvement in outcomes may be more valuable than a therapy provided to all HHF patients that provided only a 5% improvement in outcomes. The number needed to treat to see an improved outcome is 5 and 20 for the targeted and general therapy, respectively. A more targeted approach would spare the majority of patients from the possible toxicities, costs, and burden of an additional therapy while also delivering the treatment to patients most likely to benefit. Designing effective trials with a more personalized approach may be aided by a bayesian adaptive trial design[35] that makes use of initial data and augments with data accumulated during the trial to identify and tailor therapies for subgroups that are more likely to benefit. In doing so, inefficiencies of megatrials may be able to be reduced, therapies (eg, different dosing regimens) more stringently evaluated, and patients identified who are likely to benefit the most, improving return on investments for payers.

Study Execution

Beyond trial design, study execution needs to improve. Many participating centers provide marginal quality and there is often limited knowledge of the center, its ability to recruit and execute the protocol, and the characteristics of the patients it enrolls. There are differences in patient characteristics and outcomes among various regions within a trial,[36,37] the reasons for which and its impact on the overall study are unclear. Patient characteristics and outcomes in a trial are also related to the intensity of recruitment.[38] Data suggest factors such as location of a center and number of patients enrolled relate to outcomes, thereby necessitating evaluation of each center. This may be aided by a pretrial registry characterizing the patients that the center enrolls so that the right patients for a given intervention and study protocol can be identified. This registry could also serve as a screening tool for centers. It could help identify quality centers that are capable of enrolling appropriate patients in reasonable numbers and executing the protocol correctly. Knowledge of participating centers through a registry can facilitate identification of fewer centers enrolling more patients and eliminating those that enroll few,[39] allocating resources to developing operational capabilities of effective centers to achieve the desired timely enrollment and not to frequent site visits to low-enrolling centers. Efforts spent early to create simple user-friendly protocols can facilitate study execution.

Stakeholder Cooperation

To develop therapies that reach the patients, cooperation among all stakeholders is imperative. Early and frequent communication can help improve therapeutic development. Ultimately, the regulators and payers determine what reaches patients; understanding their priorities should be part of the initial steps in developing therapies. Early communication with regulatory bodies and payers regarding endpoints for approval and reimbursement may guide which endpoints to test and how to design trials. Payers want efficacy, cost-effectiveness, accountability, and access. With the use of electronic medical records, payers expect using technology to reduce costs and improve outcomes, potentially through earlier detection of risk.[40] The shift in reimbursements to including metrics of success reflects the value

payers have in accountability. Payers want to see therapies that can be scaled for a community, market, or health care system. Cooperation can improve trial execution, which industry has recognized in creating TranCelerate BioPharma, a nonprofit organization made up of 10 pharmaceutical developers with initial goals of standardizing the recording of data and creating a standard Web portal to ease communication with sites.[41] By working together from initial stages, therapies can move swiftly from development, to translational and research, to regulatory approval, and to patients.

SUMMARY

HHF signifies a high-risk state with an unmet need and potential for new therapies to improve outcomes. There is considerable diversity of both the underlying pathophysiology and the patients involved. HHF is associated with an unacceptably high postdischarge mortality and rehospitalization rates. The astronomical costs associated with HHF have added demands from society, government, and payers to improve outcomes. With more than a decade of efforts at developing therapies, however, this heterogeneous group of patients is still treated with standard, homogenous therapies that are not preventing their rapid deterioration. Most of the research effort has either focused on acute phases of HHF improving short-term symptoms or long-term therapies have been targeted to chronic stable HF patients, where outcomes are not as disparate as among HHF patients. Thus it is imperative to identify HHF as a distinct entity and target long-term outcomes among these patients by improving trial design and mechanistic understanding of a potential therapy and by identifying the right patient population. Trials should be designed targeting in-hospital initiation of intervention that is continued postdischarge and should move away from megatrials to test more personalized approaches. Trial execution can be improved with a pretrial registry and a better selection of clinical sites, which can be catalyzed by cooperation and communication early and often between involved parties. These efforts may help ensure that studies are designed and executed better so that promising therapies are not dismissed and effective drugs or devices can be translated from initial development to wide-scale delivery efficiently and safely. In doing so, all parties can witness return on their investment in effort, time, and money. Most importantly, with coordinated and committed efforts in the development of new therapies, improvements that matter may be seen in outcomes for patients with HHF.

ACKNOWLEDGMENTS

Felipe Aguel and Preston Dunnmon represented the Food and Drug Administration's point of view at this panel session at the Heart Failure Society of America's Annual Scientific Meeting.

DISCLOSURES

M. Gheorghiade, MD: consultant to Abbott Laboratories, Astellas, Astra Zeneca, Bayer Schering Pharma AG, CorThera, Cytokinetics, DebioPharm SA, Errekappa Terapeutici, GlaxoSmithKline, Johnson & Johnson, Medtronic, Merck, Novartis Pharma AG, Otsuka Pharmaceuticals, Pericor Therapeutics, Protein Design Laboratories, Sanofi-Aventis, Sigma Tau, and Solvay Pharmaceuticals. J. Butler, MD, MPH: consultant to Cardio-MEMS, Bayer HealthCare, Trevena, Ono Pharma, and Gambro; research support from Medtronic, National Institutes of Health, and Amgen. S. Taylor, RPh, MBA: employed by Geisinger Health System. S. Kupfer, MD: employed by Takeda Global Research and Development Center, Inc. F. Misselwitz, MD, PhD: employed by Bayer Health-Care. G.C. Fonarow, MD: research support from Medtronic, Novartis, and Gambro. A.N. Shah, MD; M. Vaduganathan, MD, MPH; G.M.C. Rosano, MD, PhD; and A. Sharma, MD: None.

REFERENCES

1. Askoxylakis V, Thieke C, Pleger ST, et al. Long-term survival of cancer patients compared to heart failure and stroke: a systematic review. BMC Cancer 2010; 10:105.
2. Heidenreich PA, Trogdon JG, Khavjou OA, et al. Forecasting the future of cardiovascular disease in the United States: a policy statement from the American Heart Association. Circulation 2011;123: 933–44.
3. Roger VL, Go AS, Lloyd-Jones DM, et al. Heart disease and stroke statistics–2012 update: a report from the American Heart Association. Circulation 2012;125:e2–220.
4. Chen J, Normand SL, Wang Y, et al. National and regional trends in heart failure hospitalization and mortality rates for Medicare beneficiaries, 1998-2008. JAMA 2011;306:1669–78.
5. Gheorghiade M, Abraham WT, Albert NM, et al. Systolic blood pressure at admission, clinical characteristics, and outcomes in patients hospitalized with acute heart failure. JAMA 2006;296:2217–26.
6. Fonarow GC, Peterson ED. Heart failure performance measures and outcomes: real or illusory gains. JAMA 2009;302:792–4.
7. Epstein AM, Jha AK, Orav EJ. The relationship between hospital admission rates and rehospitalizations. N Engl J Med 2011;365:2287–95.
8. Setoguchi S, Stevenson LW, Schneeweiss S. Repeated hospitalizations predict mortality in the community population with heart failure. Am Heart J 2007;154:260–6.
9. Wilcox JE, Fonarow GC, Yancy CW, et al. Factors associated with improvement in ejection fraction in clinical practice among patients with heart failure: findings from IMPROVE HF. Am Heart J 2012;163: 49–56.e2.
10. Axon RN, Williams MV. Hospital readmission as an accountability measure. JAMA 2011;305:504–5.
11. Korves C, Eldar-Lissai A, McHale J, et al. Resource utilization and costs following hospitalization of patients with chronic heart failure in the US. J Med Econ 2012;15:925–37.
12. Butler J, Fonarow GC, Gheorghiade M. Strategies and opportunities for drug development in heart failure. JAMA 2013;309:1593–4.
13. Gheorghiade M, Pang PS, O'Connor CM, et al. Clinical development of pharmacologic agents for acute heart failure syndromes: a proposal for a mechanistic translational phase. Am Heart J 2011;161: 224–32.
14. Gheorghiade M, Pang PS. Acute heart failure syndromes. J Am Coll Cardiol 2009;53:557–73.
15. Gottlieb SS. Renal effects of adenosine A1-receptor antagonists in congestive heart failure. Drugs 2001; 61:1387–93.
16. Gottlieb SS, Brater DC, Thomas I, et al. BG9719 (CVT-124), an A1 adenosine receptor antagonist, protects against the decline in renal function observed with diuretic therapy. Circulation 2002; 105:1348–53.
17. Gottlieb SS, Skettino SL, Wolff A, et al. Effects of BG9719 (CVT-124), an A1-adenosine receptor antagonist, and furosemide on glomerular filtration rate and natriuresis in patients with congestive heart failure. J Am Coll Cardiol 2000;35:56–9.
18. Massie BM, O'Connor CM, Metra M, et al. Rolofylline, an adenosine A1-receptor antagonist, in acute heart failure. N Engl J Med 2010;363:1419–28.
19. Gottlieb SS, Abraham W, Butler J, et al. The prognostic importance of different definitions of worsening renal function in congestive heart failure. J Card Fail 2002;8:136–41.
20. Goldenberg I, Gillespie J, Moss AJ, et al. Long-term benefit of primary prevention with an implantable cardioverter-defibrillator: an extended 8-year follow-up study of the Multicenter Automatic Defibrillator Implantation Trial II. Circulation 2010;122: 1265–71.

21. Mebazaa A, Pang PS, Tavares M, et al. The impact of early standard therapy on dyspnoea in patients with acute heart failure: the URGENT-dyspnoea study. Eur Heart J 2010;31:832–41.

22. Teerlink JR. Dyspnea as an end point in clinical trials of therapies for acute decompensated heart failure. Am Heart J 2003;145:S26–33.

23. West RL, Hernandez AF, O'Connor CM, et al. A review of dyspnea in acute heart failure syndromes. Am Heart J 2010;160:209–14.

24. Pang PS, Cleland JG, Teerlink JR, et al. A proposal to standardize dyspnoea measurement in clinical trials of acute heart failure syndromes: the need for a uniform approach. Eur Heart J 2008;29:816–24.

25. Collins SP, Pang PS, Lindsell CJ, et al. International variations in the clinical, diagnostic, and treatment characteristics of emergency department patients with acute heart failure syndromes. Eur J Heart Fail 2010;12:1253–60.

26. Konstam MA, Gheorghiade M, Burnett JC Jr, et al. Effects of oral tolvaptan in patients hospitalized for worsening heart failure: the EVEREST Outcome Trial. JAMA 2007;297:1319–31.

27. Gheorghiade M, Konstam MA, Burnett JC Jr, et al. Short-term clinical effects of tolvaptan, an oral vasopressin antagonist, in patients hospitalized for heart failure: the EVEREST Clinical Status Trials. JAMA 2007;297:1332–43.

28. Gheorghiade M, Adams KF, Cleland JG, et al. Phase III clinical trial end points in acute heart failure syndromes: a virtual roundtable with the Acute Heart Failure Syndromes International Working Group. Am Heart J 2009;157:957–70.

29. Gheorghiade M, Zannad F, Sopko G, et al. Acute heart failure syndromes: current state and framework for future research. Circulation 2005;112: 3958–68.

30. Publication Committee for the VMAC Investigators (Vasodilatation in the Management of Acute CHF). Intravenous nesiritide vs nitroglycerin for treatment of decompensated congestive heart failure: a randomized controlled trial. JAMA 2002;287: 1531–40.

31. Cuffe MS, Califf RM, Adams KF Jr, et al. Short-term intravenous milrinone for acute exacerbation of chronic heart failure: a randomized controlled trial. JAMA 2002;287:1541–7.

32. McMurray JJ, Teerlink JR, Cotter G, et al. Effects of tezosentan on symptoms and clinical outcomes in patients with acute heart failure: the VERITAS randomized controlled trials. JAMA 2007;298:2009–19.

33. Mebazaa A, Nieminen MS, Packer M, et al. Levosimendan vs. dobutamine for patients with acute decompensated heart failure: the SURVIVE Randomized Trial. JAMA 2007;297:1883–91.

34. O'Connor CM, Starling RC, Hernandez AF, et al. Effect of nesiritide in patients with acute decompensated heart failure. N Engl J Med 2011;365:32–43.

35. Collins SP, Lindsell CJ, Pang PS, et al. Bayesian adaptive trial design in acute heart failure syndromes: moving beyond the mega trial. Am Heart J 2012;164:138–45.

36. Blair JE, Zannad F, Konstam MA, et al. Continental differences in clinical characteristics, management, and outcomes in patients hospitalized with worsening heart failure results from the EVEREST (Efficacy of Vasopressin Antagonism in Heart Failure: Outcome Study with Tolvaptan) program. J Am Coll Cardiol 2008;52:1640–8.

37. Atherton JJ, Hayward CS, Wan Ahmad WA, et al. Patient characteristics from a regional multicenter database of acute decompensated heart failure in Asia Pacific (ADHERE International-Asia Pacific). J Card Fail 2012;18:82–8.

38. Gheorghiade M, Vaduganathan M, Greene SJ, et al. Site selection in global clinical trials in patients hospitalized for heart failure: perceived problems and potential solutions. Heart Fail Rev 2012. [Epub ahead of print].

39. Butler J, Subacius H, Vaduganathan M, et al. Relationship between clinical trial site enrollment with participant characteristics, protocol completion, and outcomes: insights from the EVEREST (Efficacy of Vasopressin Antagonism in Heart Failure: Outcome Study with Tolvaptan) Trial. J Am Coll Cardiol 2013;61(5):571–9.

40. Wu J, Roy J, Stewart WF. Prediction modeling using EHR data: challenges, strategies, and a comparison of machine learning approaches. Med Care 2010; 48:S106–13, 21.

41. Pollack A. Drug makers join efforts in research. The New York Times, September 19, 2012. Available at: http://www.nytimes.com/2012/09/20/health/drug-makers-in-joint-effort-to-streamlineresearch. Accessed December 13, 2012.

Initial Management of Patients with Acute Heart Failure

Gregory J. Fermann, MD[a],*, Sean P. Collins, MD, MSc[b]

KEYWORDS

- Acute heart failure • Diagnosis • Risk stratification • Treatment • Emergency care

KEY POINTS

- More than 80% of patients with acute decompensated heart failure (ADHF) present to the emergency department (ED), and significant pressures exist to manage these patients efficiently in the acute-care environment.
- Most patients with ADHF present to the ED with worsening of chronic heart failure (HF); some may present with undifferentiated dyspnea and new-onset HF, whereas others have significant comorbidities that complicate diagnosis and treatment.
- Although physical examination, electrocardiography, chest radiography, natriuretic peptides, and necrosis markers remain the cornerstones of diagnosis, the role of bedside ultrasonography will continue to expand.
- Treatment of patients with ADHF is prioritized based on vital signs and presenting phenotype.
- Vasodilators and loop diuretics remain the mainstay in initial therapy, although newer vasoactive compounds may be available soon.
- Risk stratification of patients, particularly those who may show low-risk features, is the subject of ongoing evaluation.
- Disposition of patients to areas other than a monitored inpatient bed, such as an ED-based observation unit, may prove effective in the ever-changing health care climate.

INTRODUCTION

Acute decompensated heart failure (ADHF) represents the primary admitting diagnoses for more than 1 million patients per year. As the most common cause for admission in patients older than 65 years, visits because of ADHF have tripled in the last 3 decades.[1,2] Given an increasing aged population and improved outcomes in sudden cardiac death and acute myocardial infarction, the trajectory of increasing ADHF presentations to acute-care institutions will undoubtedly continue.[3] The in-hospital mortality of these patients is 5% and has decreased 40% over the past decade. Mean length of stay in hospital is 5 to 6 days and has decreased over the same period. However, readmission rates remain unchanged at 25% within 30 days and 50% within 6 to 12 months. Mortality has persistently been 5% to 10% at 30 days after hospital discharge and 20% to 40% 6 to 12 months after hospital discharge.[4–6]

Disclosures: Dr Collins has received research support from NIH/NHLBI K23HL085387, Medtronic, Radiometer, and Cardiorentis. He has also been a consultant for Novartis, Trevena, The Medicines Company, and BRAHMS. Dr Fermann has received research support from Medtronic, Radiometer, Cardiorentis, Nanodetection Technologies, and Cubist Pharmaceuticals. He is also a Consultant to Pfizer.

[a] Department of Emergency Medicine, University of Cincinnati, 231 Albert Sabin Way, ML 0769, Cincinnati, OH 45267, USA; [b] Department of Emergency Medicine, Vanderbilt University, 703 Oxford House (4700), 1313 21st Avenue South, Nashville, TN 37232-4700, USA
* Corresponding author.
E-mail address: gregory.fermann@uc.edu

Heart Failure Clin 9 (2013) 291–301
http://dx.doi.org/10.1016/j.hfc.2013.04.004
1551-7136/13/$ – see front matter © 2013 Elsevier Inc. All rights reserved.

Given the staggering disease burden and recidivism, the cost of ADHF is substantial. Direct and inherent costs for treating ADHF were expected to total 34.8 billion dollars in 2008, with 75% of ADHF-related costs being incurred in the first 48 hours after presentation.[7] Because more than 80% of patients with ADHF present to the emergency department (ED), significant pressures exist to manage these patients efficiently in the acute-care environment.[8] Selected patients may be eligible to receive care for ADHF in an observation unit (OU), which may provide a safe and effective means to lower costs by providing an alternative to an inpatient stay.[9] Previous studies have suggested that more than 50% of such patients are appropriate for a brief period of observation and treatment aimed at avoiding inpatient admission. However, the limited data in those discharged directly from the ED suggest that they have a high rate of adverse events.[10,11] Thus, the decision to admit an ED patient with ADHF is often not based on acute severity of disease. Instead, it is largely a function of medical comorbidities and the uncertainty regarding near-term events. Thus, a safe alternative to hospital admission is a critical unmet need.

Although the hemodynamically unstable patient with ADHF poses significant challenges to the cardiologist and emergency physician, these presentations account for less than 5% of the total population with ADHF.[4,12] Most are symptomatic yet hemodynamically stable, at least initially. The management of this patient population requires a balance between supporting hemodynamic stability, improving signs and symptoms, and decision making to minimize morbidity and mortality. Although it is easy for the emergency medicine (EM) physician to identify those patients who are hemodynamically unstable or critically ill, it is sometimes difficult to identify those patients with ADHF who require hospitalization versus those who can be discharged after a brief period of observation. Because there are few data to aid EM physicians when trying to identify low-risk patients who are safe for ED discharge, risk stratification in this vulnerable patient population is the subject of ongoing study.[13–16]

The initial evaluation of patients who present with signs and symptoms of ADHF focuses on increasing the degree of diagnostic certainty that ADHF is present rather than the myriad of other causes of acute dyspnea. Symptom relief is the therapeutic focus after initial stabilization. Risk stratification occurs concurrently with diagnosis and treatment and can guide the decision of where to best triage patients, such as the intensive care unit (ICU), telemetry, or observation. In this review,

diagnostic and treatment modalities, clinical considerations, risk stratification tools, and disposition options in patients presenting to the ED with ADHF are discussed.

DIAGNOSIS
History

Patients with ADHF often present with dyspnea. Dyspnea on exertion, paroxysmal nocturnal dyspnea (PND), and orthopnea, although common, are not highly predictive of ADHF. In a large meta-analysis examining the predictors of ADHF,[17] PND and orthopnea have intermediate likelihood ratios (LRs) of 2.6 and 2.2, respectively, for a diagnosis of ADHF. Historical features such as lower extremity edema, fatigue, previous episodes of ADHF, recent medication changes, dietary indiscretion, or modifications are often routinely asked about. Duration of symptoms often gives subtle cues to the phenotype of the heart failure (HF). Signs of volume overload and peripheral edema with an onset over days to weeks are often suggestive of gradual worsening of HF with reduced ejection fraction (HFREF).[18] Poorly controlled blood pressure (BP), arrhythmias, or acute coronary syndrome (ACS) may cause more rapid decompensation.

Physical Examination

Vital signs can be helpful in determining the cause of ADHF as well as guiding initial management and therapy. Patients with diastolic dysfunction and HF with preserved ejection fraction (HFPEF) often present with high BP.[19] However, both those with systolic and diastolic dysfunction can present with increased BP.[20] Bradycardia might implicate heart block, drug toxicity (specifically digoxin), and electrolyte abnormalities as precipitants of the ADHF presentation. The physical examination findings most suggestive of ADHF include a third heart sound (S3), and jugular venous distention (JVD). Although bibasilar rales and peripheral edema are helpful, they are less specific for ADHF. An S3 gallop and JVD have an LR of 11 and 5.1, respectively, for ADHF, whereas rales and peripheral edema have an LR of 2.8 and 2.3, respectively.[17]

Chest Radiography

Cardiomegaly, cephalization, interstitial edema, alveolar edema, or pleural effusions are all found in ADHF. Interstitial edema is well correlated with ADHF, with an LR of 12.0.[17] Cardiomegaly and pleural effusions, with LRs of 3.3 and 3.2, may be findings that are more common in chronic HF than AHDF. ED patients with ADHF have no radiographic findings of congestion in 13% to 15% of cases.[21]

Natriuretic Peptides

Natriuretic peptides (NP), released from myocytes secondary to myocardial stretch and increasing end diastolic pressures, have been found to be useful as a diagnostic tool in patients in whom there is still uncertainty after traditional testing.[22,23] Increased NP levels are indicators of both the presence and severity of illness. The Breathing Not Properly trial suggested that brain NP (BNP) levels can be used to increase diagnostic accuracy when added to clinical judgment. The dyspneic patient with a plasma BNP level of less than 100 pg/dL or N-terminal (NT)-proBNP of less than 300 pg/dL is unlikely to have ADHF. BNP levels of greater than 500 pg/dL have 90% specificity in the prediction of ADHF as the cause of dyspnea. Of the 26.4% of patients with gray zone BNP levels between 100 and 500 pg/dL, two-thirds (16.5%) may still have HF as the cause of dyspnea.[23] NT-proBNP has also shown a similar diagnostic usefulness.[24] In certain patient populations, the NPs can be falsely high or low. Both are falsely increased in renal insufficiency, NT-proBNP more than BNP.[25] Obese patients tend to have falsely lower BNP levels because of BNP metabolism in adipose tissue.[18]

Necrosis Markers

Serial monitoring of cardiac necrosis biomarkers, especially cardiac troponin (cTn), is recommended for diagnostic and prognostic purposes. Patients with ADHF with elevation of cTn have higher mortality than those with nondetectable cTn. The magnitude of the increase is not specified. Results from data from a large ADHF registry using troponin I levels of greater than 1 μg/L and troponin T levels of 0.1 μg/L found an independent association with in-hospital mortality.[26] Outcome studies of lower-level troponin increases using ultrasensitive methods are ongoing. In HFPEF with ADHF, minor myocardial damage, defined as increases of cTn of more than 0.02 ng/mL, were found in 44% of patients.[27] Patients with an increased Tn were also found to have higher markers of disease severity, such as lower ejection fraction (EF), higher serum creatinine level, higher NP level, and higher 6-month event rates.[27]

Electrocardiography

A 12-lead electrocardiogram (ECG) is important to identify treatable conditions such as cardiac ischemia and arrhythmias. Atrial fibrillation in the setting of dyspnea has been the most studied arrhythmia in patients with ADHF.[17] However, new T-wave changes or any abnormal ECG can also be associated with ADHF. A normal ECG decreases the likelihood of ADHF.[17]

Evolving Diagnostic Strategies

Echocardiography was once considered a test that was obtained during inpatient admission. However, with the introduction of portable high-resolution ultrasound devices and advanced training for EM physicians, bedside echocardiography in the ED continues to evolve. After initial management and stabilization of the patient with suspected ADHF, limited bedside echocardiography can give the clinician information about cardiovascular pathophysiology. The use of mitral valve E point septal separation (EPSS) in M-mode ultrasonography has been established as an option to assess for reduced EF. A sensitivity of 87% for detecting an abnormal EF at a cutoff of greater than 7 mm has been reported.[28] EM residents (PGY3/4) were able to obtain EPSS measurements that closely correlate with the visual estimates of EF made by experienced sonographers.[29]

Rapid assessment for increased central venous pressure (CVP) as a marker of right heart congestion can also be assessed. An inferior vena cava greater than 2 cm or collapsibility index of less than 50% indicates increased CVP. In the absence of significant pulmonary disease, this factor has been found to be highly correlated with pulmonary capillary wedge pressure.[30] Measuring diastolic parameters can identify decreased left ventricular compliance and diastolic dysfunction. An early/late ratio greater than 2 indicates decreased left ventricular compliance and has been shown to be 100% sensitive and specific in predicting a left ventricular end diastolic pressure greater than 20 mm Hg.[31]

Comet tail artifacts, ultrasonographic evidence of B-lines, are additional diagnostic findings readily assessed by the EM physician using bedside ultrasonography (Fig. 1). B-lines arise from water-thickened interlobular septa at the pleural line. Assessment of B-lines can help differentiate between cardiogenic and noncardiogenic causes of dyspnea. The technique involves assessment of the anterior and lateral chest wall from the second to fifth intercostal spaces.[32] Three or more B-lines in 1 viewing field are considered a positive finding for pulmonary edema. In one study[33] evaluating 149 patients who presented with acute dyspnea, ultrasonographic B-lines were found in 93 of the 122 patients who were found to have a

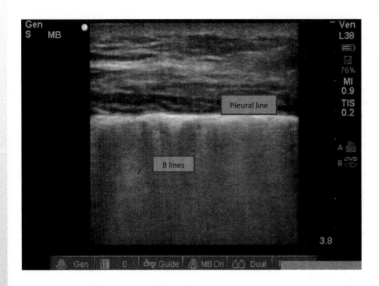

Fig. 1. Ultrasound B-lines (comet tails). (*Courtesy of* Laura Kress, RDCS, RVT, Cincinnati, OH.)

cardiogenic cause of dyspnea. Whereas the negative predictive value was superior for NT-proBNP (100%) over B-lines (45%), the positive predictive value for B-lines (97%) was marginally better than NT-proBNP (92%).

THERAPY
General Approach to Therapy

ADHF therapy as applied to the ED setting can be conceptualized as a 2-fold approach: symptom relief and initiation of inpatient therapy. Although most patients known to have HF have been prescribed approved medications as outpatients, ED care pathways most often involve restarting the medications that have been missed or adjusting dosages on medications that the patient is are already taking. Symptom relief is often tailored to treat the presenting clinical profile.

Symptom relief

Non–potassium-sparing diuretics (ie, loop diuretics) are the mainstay of symptom therapy in ADHF. Although the goal of fluid removal remains primary in initial inpatient therapy, electrolyte imbalances, renal dysfunction, and alteration of neurohormonal balance can develop with high furosemide doses. The DOSE (Diuretic Optimization Strategies Evaluation) study[34] randomized patients to low-dose (same as oral daily dose) or high-dose (2.5 times oral daily dose) parenteral furosemide therapy. Using a factorial design, patients were also randomized to bolus (twice daily) or continuous administration. Results show a trend toward greater symptom relief in the high-dose group, with secondary improvement in volume loss and decreased weight. The median change

of serum creatinine level was 0.06 mg/dL and 0.01 mg/dL for the high-dose and low-dose protocols, respectively. Unlike previous studies, continuous infusion was not superior to intermittent bolus therapy. Patients were enrolled in this study long after ED presentation, making extrapolation of these data to the ED patient difficult. Despite the obvious clinical usefulness of diuretic use, clinicians should be aware of the possible association of diuretic use as a marker of increased risk.[4] The use of ultrafiltration has not been adequately studied in the ED setting to advocate routine use. Thus far, trials of vasopressin antagonists have failed to show significant improvement in ADHF symptoms.[35]

Nitroglycerin is a potent arteriole and venous vasodilator and reduces both afterload and preload rapidly. Because it can be delivered by several routes, such as intravenous, sublingual, topical, spray, and tablet, nitroglycerin remains a popular first-line therapy for symptom relief in patients without low BP.[21] The intravenous form can be titrated based on BP and symptom response, but often mandates admission to a critical care bed. Morphine has historically been used in ADHF because of its mild venodilator activity, preload reduction, and anxiolysis. The data supporting its use have been anecdotal and were contradicted by reports describing increased rates of endotracheal intubation, ICU admission, and prolonged hospital stay. Recent data from the ADHERE registry (Acute Decompensated Heart Failure National Registry) found an association between morphine use and increased in-hospital mortality.[36] Given these reports, if morphine is used, it should be in a judicious manner.

Nesiritide was approved for the treatment of ADHF in the United States in 2001. Although it improves hemodynamics and dyspnea,[37,38] pooled data raised concerns over worsening renal function and increased mortality.[39] The safety and efficacy of nesiritide was studied in the ASCEND-HF (Acute Study of Clinical Effectiveness of Nesiritide in Decompensated Heart Failure) trial,[40] a double-blind, placebo-controlled, multinational trial. Results suggest that it is safe, but did not meet the prespecified end point for improvement of dyspnea. The use of nesiritide in OUs has been evaluated by the PROACTION (Prospective Randomized Outcomes study of Acutely decompensated CHF Treated Initially as Outpatients with Nesiritide) trial. There were no differences in adverse outcomes between standard care and nesiritide. The nesiritide group was shown to have fewer hospital days (2.5 days vs 6.5 days; $P = .03$) in the month after administration.[41,42]

A recent randomized study of relaxin in ADHF suggests this therapy may safely improve dyspnea, minimize ongoing myocardial and renal injury, and perhaps improve long-term events.[43] This study enrolled patients earlier than previous ADHF studies, with a minimum systolic BP of 125 mm Hg, which may be an explanation for the promising results. Early enrollment suggests that this therapy may have a role in ED patients with ADHF, but further study is necessary.[44]

Although the use of angiotensin-converting enzyme (ACE) inhibitors in chronic HF management is well supported, their role in the acute setting is less clear.[45] The use of enalaprilat, an intravenous ACE inhibitor, in ADHF is a level C recommendation by the American College of Emergency Physicians, and is not recommended by the European Society of Cardiology.[46] It has been shown to improve hemodynamics in small studies,[47] but has not been definitively evaluated in a large-scale trial. Nitroprusside is a potent systemic and pulmonary vasodilator, which requires invasive monitoring and frequent titration, and is not well suited to an ED environment. Positive inotropes with properties favorable for patients with ADHF with low output states, like dobutamine, milrinone, and levosimendan (available in Europe) are useful in only a few patients who present with ADHF and signs of impaired perfusion.

Patients who present with ADHF may require oxygen supplementation. The amount of oxygen that must be administered after initial therapy is often a key triage data point. After initial steps at symptom relief, patients can be titrated down to nasal cannula administration that can be easily managed in a non-ICU environment. Ventilatory support through endotracheal intubation or noninvasive ventilation (NIV) mandates ICU admission. NIV support either through continuous positive airway pressure support or bilevel positive airway pressure may reduce the need for intubation, shorten ICU stay, and reduce cost but likely has no impact on mortality.[48,49] If patients can be weaned off NIV in the ED, transferring their care to an OU or telemetry floor can be considered if other parameters are met. Hyperoxia should be avoided.[50]

Implementation of outpatient therapies

Depending on specific ADHF pathways, ED management of this patient population may include initiation of inpatient therapies in collaboration with the inpatient team of cardiologists or hospitalists. β-Blockers improve survival in HF and are a mainstay in outpatient treatment. There was controversy as to whether these agents should be withheld during acute exacerbations. Most recent guidelines suggest that patients taking long-term evidenced-based β-blockers (carvedilol, metoprolol CR/XL, or bisoprolol) should continue them even in ADHF unless hypoperfusion is present. Dosages can be down titrated or held if hypotension or bradycardia arises.[51,52] ACE inhibitors and angiotensin receptor blockers (ARBs) are standard therapy in chronic HF management. They improve symptoms, decrease morbidity and mortality, and slow disease progression in patients with reduced left ventricular EF (EF <40%).[46] They should be continued in those patients who are taking them chronically. Because they are contraindicated in patients with hyperkalemia (K >5.5 mmol/L), as well as pregnancy, symptomatic hypotension, bilateral renal artery stenosis, or angioedema, they should be given after potassium levels and renal function have been checked. ADHF protocols should have a standardized approach to β-blocker and ACE inhibitor/ARB delivery, with careful documentation of contraindications or intolerances. Oral digoxin has been historically used to improve hemodynamics and symptoms with chronic use, and when added to diuretic and ACE inhibitor, can decrease hospitalization.[53] Intravenous digoxin use in ADHF is less well studied.

Tailored Therapy

The clinical profile is initially described based on the presenting hemodynamics; hypertensive, normotensive, and hypotensive. Patients who present with increased systolic BP (>140 mm Hg) have a predominance of pulmonary congestion, clinically or radiographically, with milder signs of systemic congestion. The onset of symptoms is often over 24 to 48 hours, and more than 50% of patients present with systolic BP greater than 140 mm Hg.[21,54] These patients often have HFPEF and may present with acute, severe dyspnea and diaphoresis. Although the treating clinician may entertain delivering ventilatory support until other treatment modalities take effect, these patients often respond dramatically with aggressive, timely intervention. The treatment focuses on reducing afterload with vasodilators such as nitrates (sublingual, intravenous, or topical), hydralazine (intravenous), and ACE inhibitors. Although loop diuretics are often used, symptoms in these patients are often caused by rapid fluid shifts into the pulmonary vascular bed and are not necessarily caused by increased whole-body edema.[55,56]

By contrast, patients with HFREF may present with normal or moderately increased BP, with systemic congestion developing over days to weeks, with few signs or symptoms of pulmonary congestion. These patients often respond to more aggressive diuresis and may not require vasodilators acutely. The optimal diuretic regimen is the subject of recent investigation.[34] A few (<8%) who present with low BP (<90 mm Hg) as a result of very low cardiac output, superimposed infection, or hypovolemia and decreased renal perfusion, or in cardiogenic shock, are unique therapeutic challenges.[57] These patients should be triaged as quickly as possible to the ICU for advanced medical and mechanical therapies.

Overall, the management of the patient with ADHF in the ED is based on the physician's ability to identify critical elements of the patient's history and presentation to administer appropriate treatment and determine disposition. **Table 1** shows the balance of considerations that the ED physician must consider to appropriately manage the patient with ADHF and also highlights the complexity and heterogeneity of ADHF presentations.[21,58]

Table 1 Clinical considerations	
1. BP	**Associated Findings and Strategies**
Hypotensive (<5%)	Fluids Inotropes ICU admit
Normotensive	Insidious onset (days, weeks) Diuretics ± vasodilators ED observation vs telemetry floor
Hypertensive (~50%)	Acute onset (24–72 h) Vasodilator, diuretics ED observation vs telemetry floor
2. Comorbidities	**Associated Findings**
Chronic renal insufficiency	Chronically increased BNP, Difficult diuresis
Obstructive pulmonary disorder	Wheezing on physical examination
Obesity	Low BNP, Difficult physical examination
3. Clinical Severity Present in extremis with pulmonary edema Insidious presentation	
4. Heart Rate and Rhythm Rapid atrial fibrillation/flutter: consider β-blocker vs calcium channel blocker Bradycardia: consider heart block, drug toxicity, electrolyte abnormality	
5. Precipitants Diet Medicine ACS, arrhythmia	
6. De novo vs acute exacerbation of chronic HF De novo: broad differential, consider ACS/arrhythmia Chronic HF: consider precipitants, current medications	

RISK STRATIFICATION

The patient who presents in cardiogenic shock caused by ADHF is at substantial risk of morbidity and mortality. However, most patients who present to the ED with dyspnea caused by ADHF and gradual worsening of chronic HF are not critically ill. This group also has substantial risk of immediate and short-term adverse events. One prospective cohort study[59] showed that triage physicians overestimate the probability of severe complications in the patient with ADHF and as a result tend to overuse critical care resources for admission. Although the predominant consideration in risk stratification as it applies to the

emergency care of the patient with ADHF is short-term event rates, no gold standard time frame exists. The events rates are often conceptualized by emergency physicians as immediate adverse events (those within 7 days or within the index hospitalization) and short-term (those events occurring within 30 days of ED presentation). Several studies have identified markers of short-term risk. They include increased blood urea nitrogen (BUN) or creatinine levels, hyponatremia, ECG evidence of myocardial ischemia, increased BNP, increased cTn, or low BP.[54,60,61] However, because 80% of all patients with ADHF are admitted to the hospital and often to a monitored bed, the identification of the high-risk patient has less impact on emergency decision making than identification of the low-risk patient. The lack of high-risk features does not identify a patient who is low risk.

Given the reluctance of US clinicians to discharge patients directly from the ED, is there evidence supporting the identification of a low-risk cohort? Auble and colleagues[62] aimed to derive a clinical prediction rule to identify patients with ADHF who are at low risk of death or serious medical complication based on readily available patient data in the ED. They used administrative data and a complex classification algorithm to retrospectively derive a tool that uses 21 variables to describe patients at low risk for poor outcome. This model was validated by applying this clinical prediction rule to a retrospective cohort of 8384 inpatients with a primary diagnosis of ADHF. Of this cohort, 1609 (19.2%) were identified as low risk. Of those identified as low risk, 12 (0.7%) died as inpatients, 28 (1.7%) survived after a serious hospital complication, and 47 (2.9%) died within 30 days of discharge.[62,63] This tool has yet to be studied prospectively to determine how it would augment physician decision making. A recent Canadian study also explored the use of a risk scoring system to identify high-risk patients. Using variables readily available to the emergency physicians and a novel 3-minute walk test, Stiell and colleagues[16] developed a 15-point, 10-variable scoring model. Using the serious adverse events definition of 30-day all-cause mortality, 14-day ADHF readmission, myocardial infarction, mechanical ventilation, percutaneous coronary intervention, coronary artery bypass graft, or renal replacement, the investigators describe low-risk score as follows: (score [risk%]): 0 (2.8%), 1 (5.1%), 2 (9.2%). This study is confounded by the significant practice variation in Canada, where less than 50% of patients with ADHF are admitted. Less than 10% of the cohort had a risk score of 0, categorized as low risk. This study highlights the difficulty of identifying a low-risk population and confirms the commonly accepted high-risk variables. The results of a recently completed study in a US cohort sponsored by the National Institutes of Health is forthcoming.[13]

DISPOSITION

Because clinical decision-making tools to aid in the risk stratification of the patient with ADHF are lacking, the disposition in the United States is often admission to the hospital. Given the uncertain reimbursement landscape, there are several unanswered questions in ADHF related to disposition decision making: is there a subset of patients who can be discharged safely from the ED with close follow-up? Who warrants 23-hour observation in an ED-based OU? Alternatives to admission are dependent on individual patient factors and the infrastructure of the health care system where care is being provided. Both hospital resources and outpatient resources are required for comprehensive treatment of the ED patient with ADHF. One ED disposition option is stabilization, medication adjustment, and discharge home after arranging close outpatient follow-up within the next 72 hours. One study examined the trends of early outpatient follow-up on 30-day readmission rates and found that patients discharged from an inpatient admission in hospitals with higher early follow-up rates have a lower risk of 30-day readmission.[64] This finding is specific to stabilization after an inpatient stay but may suggest similar outcomes if close follow-up were established after discharge from the ED or OU. One of the crucial factors to such a process is ensuring availability of close follow-up with either a cardiologist or primary care physician. Many patients do not have a primary care physician and rely on EDs for medication adjustment and acute treatment. This subset of patients would need to have an appointment scheduled with a new provider, possibly hindering their ability to be discharged directly from the ED or after OU management. Hospital resources dedicated to finding providers for these patients would be crucial for success.

Another alternative to ED discharge is the ED-based OU. Emergency physicians are skilled and well equipped to provide acute therapy for the first 24 to 48 hours for the patient with ADHF, thus making ED-based observation a logical and economical means to care immediately for this patient population.[8,65] OUs were identified by the Institute of Medicine as central to improving resource use and patient flow. A recent study[66] suggested that increased use of the OU has the potential to save $3.1 billion and avoid 2.4 million inpatient admissions. Appropriate OU use in ADHF management may contribute to this cost saving. The impact of hospitalization on postdischarge events has not been well elucidated.[64,67,68] For the potential 50% of patients who present with ADHF and have no high-risk features, an ED-based OU may be a safe and appropriate alternative to admission to manage these patients and facilitate early discharge.[69,70] An ED OU has the potential to provide the resources necessary to monitor BP, heart rate, urine output, and weight during a 23-hour observation period, which is also adequate time for many patients to have near-complete resolution of symptoms with standard therapy.[71] Additional diagnostic testing can also be easily arranged in on OU setting, including formal echocardiography, electrolytes, and cardiac biomarkers.

SUMMARY

The initial evaluation of patients who present to the ED with ADHF remains challenging. Because more than 80% of patients with ADHF present to the ED, significant pressures exist to manage these patients efficiently in the acute-care environment. Although most patients present with worsening of chronic HF, some may present with undifferentiated dyspnea and new-onset HF. Others have significant comorbidities that complicate both the diagnosis and treatment. Although physical examination, ECG, chest radiography, NP, and necrosis markers remain as the cornerstone of diagnosis, the role of bedside ultrasonography will continue to expand. The treatment of patients with ADHF is prioritized based on vital signs and presenting phenotype. Although vasodilators and loop diuretics remain the mainstay in initial therapy, newer vasoactive compounds may be available soon. The risk stratification of patients, particularly those who may show low-risk features, is the subject of ongoing evaluation. The disposition of patients to areas other than a monitored inpatient bed, such as an ED-based OU, may prove effective in the ever-changing health care climate.

ACKNOWLEDGMENTS

The authors wish to thank Danielle Cornwall for her assistance with the preparation of this article.

REFERENCES

1. Ahmed A, Allman RM, Fonarow GC, et al. Incident heart failure hospitalization and subsequent mortality in chronic heart failure: a propensity-matched study. J Card Fail 2008;14:211.
2. Roger VL, Go AS, Lloyd-Jones DM, et al. Heart disease and stroke statistics–2012 update: a report from the American Heart Association. Circulation 2012;125(1):e2–220.
3. Abraham WT, Fonarow GC, Albert NM, et al. Predictors of in-hospital mortality in patients hospitalized for heart failure: insights from the Organized Program to Initiate Lifesaving Treatment in Hospitalized Patients with Heart Failure (OPTIMIZE-HF). J Am Coll Cardiol 2008;52:347.
4. Fonarow GC, Abraham WT, Albert NM, et al. Association between performance measures and clinical outcomes for patients hospitalized with heart failure. JAMA 2007;297(1):61–70.
5. Fonarow GC, Abraham WT, Albert NM, et al. Factors identified as precipitating hospital admissions for heart failure and clinical outcomes: findings from OPTIMIZE-HF. Arch Intern Med 2008;168:847.
6. O'Connor CM, Abraham WT, Albert NM, et al. Predictors of mortality after discharge in patients hospitalized with heart failure: an analysis from the Organized Program to Initiate Lifesaving treatment in Hospitalized Patients with Heart Failure (OPTIMIZE-HF). Am Heart J 2008;156:662.
7. Fonarow GC. Epidemiology and risk stratification in acute heart failure. Am Heart J 2008;155:200.
8. Fermann GJ, Collins SP. Observation units in the management of acute heart failure syndromes. Curr Heart Fail Rep 2010;7(3):125–33.
9. Collins SP, Schauer DP, Gupta A, et al. Cost-effectiveness analysis of ED decision making in patients with non-high-risk heart failure. Am J Emerg Med 2009;27(3):293.
10. Lee DS, Schull MJ, Alter DA, et al. Early deaths in patients with heart failure discharged from the emergency department: a population-based analysis. Circ Heart Fail 2010;3(2):228–35.
11. Rame JE, Sheffield MA, Dries DL, et al. Outcomes after emergency department discharge with a primary diagnosis of heart failure. Am Heart J 2001; 142(4):714–9.
12. Fonarow GC, Abraham WT, Albert NM, et al. Day of admission and clinical outcomes for patients hospitalized for heart failure: findings from the Organized Program to Initiate Lifesaving Treatment in Hospitalized Patients With Heart Failure (OPTIMIZE-HF). Circ Heart Fail 2008;1(1):50–7.
13. Collins SP, Lindsell CJ, Jenkins CA, et al. Risk stratification in acute heart failure: rationale and design of the STRATIFY and DECIDE studies. Am Heart J 2012;164(6):825–34.
14. Collins SP, Lindsell CJ, Pang PS, et al. Bayesian adaptive trial design in acute heart failure syndromes: moving beyond the mega trial. Am Heart J 2012;164(2):138–45.
15. Pang PS, Jesse R, Collins SP, et al. Patients with acute heart failure in the emergency department: do they all need to be admitted? J Card Fail 2012;18(12):900–3.
16. Stiell IG, Clement CM, Brison RJ, et al. A risk scoring system to identify emergency department patients with heart failure at high risk for serious adverse events. Acad Emerg Med 2013;20(1):17–26.
17. Wang CS, FitzGerald JM, Schulzer M, et al. Does this dyspneic patient in the emergency department have congestive heart failure? JAMA 2005;294(15): 1944–56.
18. Weintraub NL, Collins SP, Pang PS, et al. Acute heart failure syndromes: emergency department presentation, treatment, and disposition: current approaches and future aims: a scientific statement from the American Heart Association. Circulation 2010;122(19):1975–96.

19. Slama M, Susic D, Varagic J, et al. Diastolic dysfunction in hypertension. Curr Opin Cardiol 2002;17(4): 368–73.
20. Chatterjee K, Massie B. Systolic and diastolic heart failure: differences and similarities. J Card Fail 2007;13(7):569–76.
21. Collins S, Storrow AB, Kirk JD, et al. Beyond pulmonary edema: diagnostic, risk stratification, and treatment challenges of acute heart failure management in the emergency department. Ann Emerg Med 2008;51(1):45–57.
22. Maisel AS, Krishnaswamy P, Nowak RM, et al. Rapid measurement of B-type natriuretic peptide in the emergency diagnosis of heart failure. N Engl J Med 2002;347(3):161–7.
23. McCullough PA, Nowak RM, McCord J, et al. B-type natriuretic peptide and clinical judgment in emergency diagnosis of heart failure: analysis from Breathing Not Properly (BNP) Multinational Study. Circulation 2002;106(4):416–22.
24. Januzzi JL Jr, Camargo CA, Anwaruddin S, et al. The N-terminal Pro-BNP investigation of dyspnea in the emergency department (PRIDE) study. Am J Cardiol 2005;95(8):948–54.
25. Lamb EJ, Vickery S, Price CP. Amino-terminal pro-brain natriuretic peptide to diagnose congestive heart failure in patients with impaired kidney function. J Am Coll Cardiol 2006;48(5):1060–1 [author reply: 1061].
26. Peacock WF IV, De Marco T, Fonarow GC, et al. Cardiac troponin and outcome in acute heart failure. N Engl J Med 2008;358:2117.
27. Perna ER, Aspromonte N, Cimbaro Canella JP, et al. Minor myocardial damage is a prevalent condition in patients with acute heart failure syndromes and preserved systolic function with long-term prognostic implications: a report from the CIAST-HF (Collaborative Italo-Argentinean Study on Cardiac Troponin T in Heart Failure) study. J Card Fail 2012;18(11):822–30.
28. Ahmadpour H, Shah AA, Allen JW, et al. Mitral E point septal separation: a reliable index of left ventricular performance in coronary artery disease. Am Heart J 1983;106(1 Pt 1):21–8.
29. Secko MA, Lazar JM, Salciccioli LA, et al. Can junior emergency physicians use E-point septal separation to accurately estimate left ventricular function in acutely dyspneic patients? Acad Emerg Med 2011;18(11):1223–6.
30. Ramasubbu K, Deswal A, Chan W, et al. Echocardiographic changes during treatment of acute decompensated heart failure: insights from the ESCAPE trial. J Card Fail 2012;18(10):792–8.
31. Channer KS, Culling W, Wilde P, et al. Estimation of left ventricular end-diastolic pressure by pulsed Doppler ultrasound. Lancet 1986; 1(8488):1005–7.
32. Picano E, Frassi F, Agricola E, et al. Ultrasound lung comets: a clinically useful sign of extravascular lung water. J Am Soc Echocardiogr 2006; 19(3):356–63.
33. Prosen G, Klemen P, Strnad M. Combination of lung ultrasound (a comet-tail sign) and N-terminal pro-brain natriuretic peptide in differentiating acute heart failure from chronic obstructive pulmonary disease and asthma as cause of acute dyspnea in prehospital emergency setting. Crit Care 2011; 15(2):R114.
34. Felker GM, Lee KL, Bull DA, et al. Diuretic strategies in patients with acute decompensated heart failure. N Engl J Med 2011;364(9):797–805.
35. Konstam MA, Gheorghiade M, Burnett JC Jr, et al. Effects of oral tolvaptan in patients hospitalized for worsening heart failure: the EVEREST Outcome Trial. JAMA 2007;297(12):1319–31.
36. Peacock WF, Hollander JE, Diercks DB, et al. Morphine and outcomes in acute decompensated heart failure: an ADHERE analysis. Emerg Med J 2008;25:205.
37. Publication Committee for the VMAC I. Intravenous nesiritide vs nitroglycerin for treatment of decompensated congestive heart failure: a randomized controlled trial. JAMA 2002;287:1531–40.
38. Peacock WF IV, Emerman CL, Silver MA, et al. Nesiritide added to standard care favorably reduces systolic blood pressure compared with standard care alone in patients with acute decompensated heart failure. Am J Emerg Med 2005;157:327.
39. Sackner-Bernstein JD, Kowalski M, Fox M, et al. Short-term risk of death after treatment with nesiritide for decompensated heart failure: a pooled analysis of randomized controlled trials. JAMA 2005;293(15):1900–5.
40. Ezekowitz JA, Hernandez AF, O'Connor CM, et al. Assessment of dyspnea in acute decompensated heart failure: insights from ASCEND-HF (Acute Study of Clinical Effectiveness of Nesiritide in Decompensated Heart Failure) on the contributions of peak expiratory flow. J Am Coll Cardiol 2012; 59(16):1441–8.
41. Peacock WF IV, Holland R, Gyarmathy R, et al. Observation unit treatment of heart failure with nesiritide: results from the proaction trial. J Emerg Med 2005;29(3):243–52.
42. Ezekowitz JA, Hernandez AF, Starling RC, et al. Standardizing care for acute decompensated heart failure in a large megatrial: the approach for the Acute Studies of Clinical Effectiveness of Nesiritide in Subjects with Decompensated Heart Failure (ASCEND-HF). Am Heart J 2009;157(2): 219–28.
43. Metra M, Cotter G, Davison BA, et al. Effect of serelaxin on cardiac, renal, and hepatic biomarkers in the Relaxin in Acute Heart Failure (RELAX-AHF)

development program: correlation with outcomes. J Am Coll Cardiol 2013;61(2):196–206.

44. Teerlink JR, Cotter G, Davison BA, et al. Serelaxin, recombinant human relaxin-2, for treatment of acute heart failure (RELAX-AHF): a randomised, placebo-controlled trial. Lancet 2013;381(9860):29–39.

45. Flaherty JD, Bax JJ, DeLuca L, et al. Acute heart failure syndromes in patients with coronary artery disease: early assessment and treatment. J Am Coll Cardiol 2009;53:254.

46. Dickstein K, Cohen-Solal A, Filippatos G, et al. ESC guidelines for the diagnosis and treatment of acute and chronic heart failure 2008: the Task Force for the Diagnosis and Treatment of Acute and Chronic Heart Failure 2008 of the European Society of Cardiology. Developed in collaboration with the Heart Failure Association of the ESC (HFA) and endorsed by the European Society of Intensive Care Medicine (ESICM). Eur Heart J 2008;29:2388.

47. Annane D, Bellissant E, Pussard E, et al. Placebo-controlled, randomized, double-blind study of intravenous enalaprilat efficacy and safety in acute cardiogenic pulmonary edema. Circulation 1996; 94(6):1316–24.

48. Vital FM, Saconato H, Ladeira MT, et al. Non-invasive positive pressure ventilation (CPAP or bilevel NPPV) for cardiogenic pulmonary edema. Cochrane Database Syst Rev 2008;(3):CD005351.

49. Masip J, Betbese AJ, Paez J, et al. Non-invasive pressure support ventilation versus conventional oxygen therapy in acute cardiogenic pulmonary edema: a randomized trial. Lancet 2000;356(9248): 2126–32.

50. Mak S, Azevedo ER, Liu PP, et al. Effect of hyperoxia on left ventricular function and filling pressures in patients with and without congestive heart failure. Chest 2001;120(2):467–73.

51. Schrock JW, Emerman CL. Observation unit management of acute decompensated heart failure. Heart Fail Clin 2009;5(1):85, vii.

52. Shah SJ, Gheorghiade M. Heart failure with preserved ejection fraction: treat now by treating comorbidities. JAMA 2008;300:431.

53. Gheorghiade M, Pang PS. Acute heart failure syndromes. J Am Coll Cardiol 2009;53(7):557–73.

54. Gheorghiade M, Abraham WT, Albert NM, et al. Systolic blood pressure at admission, clinical characteristics, and outcomes in patients hospitalized with acute heart failure. JAMA 2006;296(18): 2217–26.

55. Cotter G, Metra M, Milo-Cotter O, et al. Fluid overload in acute heart failure–re-distribution and other mechanisms beyond fluid accumulation. Eur J Heart Fail 2008;10(2):165–9.

56. Cotter G, Felker GM, Adams KF, et al. The pathophysiology of acute heart failure–is it all about fluid accumulation? Am Heart J 2008;155(1):9–18.

57. Adams KF Jr, Fonarow GC, Emerman CL, et al. Characteristics and outcomes of patients hospitalized for heart failure in the United States: rationale, design, and preliminary observations from the first 100,000 cases in the Acute Decompensated Heart Failure National Registry (ADHERE). Am Heart J 2005;149(2):209–16.

58. Gheorghiade M, Braunwald E. A proposed model for initial assessment and management of acute heart failure syndromes. JAMA 2011;305(16): 1702–3.

59. Smith WR, Poses RM, McClish DK, et al. Prognostic judgments and triage decisions for patients with acute congestive heart failure. Chest 2002;121(5): 1610–7.

60. Peacock WF, Fonarow GC, Ander DS, et al. Society of Chest Pain Centers Recommendations for the evaluation and management of the observation stay acute heart failure patient: a report from the Society of Chest Pain Centers Acute Heart Failure Committee. Crit Pathw Cardiol 2008;7(2):83–6.

61. Fonarow GC, Adams KF Jr, Abraham WT, et al. Risk stratification for in-hospital mortality in acutely decompensated heart failure: classification and regression tree analysis. JAMA 2005;293(5): 572–80.

62. Auble TE, Hsieh M, Gardner W, et al. A prediction rule to identify low-risk patients with heart failure. Acad Emerg Med 2005;12(6):514–21.

63. Hsieh M, Auble TE, Yealy DM. Validation of the acute heart failure index. Ann Emerg Med 2008; 51(1):37–44.

64. Hernandez AF, Greiner MA, Fonarow GC, et al. Relationship between early physician follow-up and 30-day readmission among Medicare beneficiaries hospitalized for heart failure. JAMA 2010; 303(17):1716–22.

65. Storrow AB, Collins SP, Lyons MS, et al. Emergency department observation of heart failure: preliminary analysis of safety and cost. Congest Heart Fail 2005;11(2):68–72.

66. Baugh CW, Venkatesh AK, Hilton JA, et al. Making greater use of dedicated hospital observation units for many short-stay patients could save $3.1 billion a year. Health Aff (Millwood) 2012;31(10): 2314–23.

67. Gheorghiade M, De Luca L, Fonarow GC, et al. Pathophysiologic targets in the early phase of acute heart failure syndromes. Am J Cardiol 2005;96(6A):11G–7G.

68. Setoguchi S, Stevenson LW, Schneeweiss S. Repeated hospitalizations predict mortality in the community population with heart failure. Am Heart J 2007;154(2):260–6.

69. Graff L, Orledge J, Radford MJ, et al. Correlation of the Agency for Health Care Policy and Research congestive heart failure admission guideline with

mortality: peer review organization voluntary hospital association initiative to decrease events (PROVIDE) for congestive heart failure. Ann Emerg Med 1999;34(4 Pt 1):429–37.

70. Collins SP, Pang PS, Fonarow GC, et al. Is hospital admission for heart failure really necessary?: the role of the emergency department and observation unit in preventing hospitalization and rehospitalization. J Am Coll Cardiol 2013;61(2):121–6.

71. Peacock WF, Fonarow GC, Ander DS, et al. Society of Chest Pain Centers recommendations for the evaluation and management of the observation stay acute heart failure patient–parts 1-6. Acute Card Care 2009;11(1):3–42.

Strategies to Prevent Postdischarge Adverse Events Among Hospitalized Patients with Heart Failure

Mitchell A. Psotka, MD, PhD[a],
John R. Teerlink, MD, FESC, FRCP(UK)[b],*

KEYWORDS

- Hospitalized heart failure • Acute heart failure • Mortality • Readmission • Adverse events

KEY POINTS

- Patients hospitalized with heart failure (HF) have poor outcomes and die primarily from cardiovascular causes; sudden cardiac death and circulatory failure each are the cause of 25% to 50% of deaths.
- Readmission of HF patients is also often due to cardiovascular causes, with HF being the single largest cause, although a significant proportion is the result of arrhythmias, cardiac ischemia, and uncontrolled hypertension.
- Noncardiovascular causes make up one-third of readmissions, with primary causes being pulmonary disease and renal dysfunction.
- Many HF readmissions are complicated by medication or behavioral noncompliance. Most current inpatient therapeutics for HF do not demonstrably improve outcomes.
- Prevention of adverse outcomes in hospitalized HF patients relies on preventing HF progression by initiating and titrating evidence-based therapy, ensuring continued adherence to that therapy, and preventing and treating patient comorbidities.

INTRODUCTION

Outcomes for hospitalized patients remain staggeringly poor, with 63% of discharged Medicare patients either readmitted or dead within 1 year.[1,2] Heart failure (HF) is the primary cause of readmission for all Medicare patients, responsible for 8.6% of all medical readmissions and 6.0% of all surgical readmissions.[1] HF is diagnosed in 1% of patients older than 65 years, and the number of hospitalizations for HF is increasing.[1,3–5] Inpatient HF mortality is poor, typically greater than 4%, however most morbidity and mortality occurs after index hospital discharge.[6,7] 12.3% of all hospitalized patients are readmitted within 30 days, including 19.6% of Medicare patients. However, hospitalized HF patients have 30-day readmission rates from 20% to 27%.[1,3,8,9] Although the HF 1-year readmission rate of 55% to 65% is similar to that of Medicare patients, this does not include the 25% to 35% mortality compared with the 7% mortality for Medicare patients.[1,2,10–14]

The poor outcomes for hospitalized HF patients are multifactorial. Hospitalization serves as a marker for generally sicker patients and is

Disclosures: J.R. Teerlink has received research grants or consulting fees from Amgen, Corthera, Cytokinetics, Merck, Novartis, Takeda, and Trevena.
[a] Department of Medicine, University of California San Francisco, 505 Parnassus Avenue, San Francisco, CA 94143, USA; [b] Section of Cardiology, San Francisco Veterans Affairs Medical Center and School of Medicine, University of California San Francisco, 111C, Building 203, Room 2A-49, 4150 Clement Street, San Francisco, CA 94121-1545, USA
* Corresponding author.
E-mail address: John.Teerlink@ucsf.edu

associated with an interconnected syndrome of deconditioning, delirium, malnutrition, and sedation.[2] The proportion of readmissions attributable to HF persists or increases over time after discharge, and past HF admissions predict both readmission and mortality.[1,3,15,16] The heightened risk of readmission dissipates slowly after discharge, suggesting that any intervention should be part of a lasting care package in the outpatient setting.[3,16] Because patients are often readmitted for reasons other than their original diagnosis, interventions that apply to multiple common medical comorbidities may be more likely to reduce overall adverse events.

DEATH AND READMISSION

The primary adverse events captured by clinical trials are mortality and rehospitalization. Typical in-hospital mortality is 3% to 8%.[6,12,14,17,18] If alive after discharge, the percentage of Medicare beneficiaries readmitted (or dead) within 1 month, 3 months, or 12 months is 19.6% (plus 3.5% dead), 34.0% (plus 5.1% dead), and 56.1% (plus 6.8% dead), respectively.[1] Nonelective hospital admission is associated with severe symptoms, reduced quality of life, poor prognosis, and significant cost. Unplanned Medicare readmissions alone accounted for an estimated $17.4 billion of the total $102.6 billion yearly Medicare expenditure in data from 2003 to 2004.[1]

Rates of death and hospital readmission among patients with HF are suboptimal worldwide (Table 1).[19] In healthier patients after their first admission for HF, 30-day mortality is 5% to 7%, 1-year mortality is 22% to 26%, and the 1-year readmission rate is 13.5% to 16.1%.[20] In typical less healthy HF patients the 1-year mortality is 25% to

Table 1
Time course of mortality and readmission in select observational studies

Authors,[Ref.] Year	Patient Population	30-d Mortality (%)	30-d Readmission (%)	1-y Mortality (%)	1-y Readmission (%)
Bhatia et al,[20] 2006	Ontario, Canada first-time admissions for HF 1999–2001	5–7	4.5–4.9 (for HF only)	22.2–25.5	13.5–16.1 (for HF only)
Jencks et al,[1] 2009	All Medicare admissions 2003–2004	3.5	19.6	6.8	56.1
Jencks et al,[1] 2009	All Medicare admissions for HF 2003–2004		26.9		
Heidenreich et al,[23] 2010	VA Medical first-time admissions for HF 2002–2006	5.0–7.1	5.6–6.1	27.7–24.3	
Kociol et al,[14] 2010	ADHERE registry HFrEF and HFpEF 2001–2006	11.2–12.2	22.1–23.7	36.0–38.3	65.8–67.9
O'Connor et al,[12] 2010	EVEREST trial HFrEF patients 2003–2006			25.5	57.6
Ross et al,[21] 2010	Medicare admissions for HF 2004–2006		23.8		
Bueno et al,[9] 2010	Medicare admissions for HF 2005–2006	10.7	20.1		
Dharmarajan et al,[3] 2013	Medicare admissions for HF 2007–2009		24.8		
Kaboli et al,[151] 2012	VA medical admissions with HF, AMI, COPD, PNA, GIB 2009–2010	4.8	15.2		
Kaboli et al,[151] 2012	VA medical admissions with HF 2009–2010		20.5		

Abbreviations: AMI, acute myocardial infarction; COPD, chronic obstructive pulmonary disease; GIB, gastrointestinal bleeding; HF, heart failure; HFpEF, HF with preserved ejection fraction; HFrEF, HF with reduced ejection fraction; PNA, pneumonia; VA, Veterans Affairs.

35%, 30-day mortality is 10%, and the 1-year readmission rate is 55% to 65%. HF with reduced ejection fraction (HFrEF) and HF with preserved ejection fraction (HFpEF) each make up 50% of hospitalized HF patients and have similarly poor outcomes.[13] In a general registry with HFrEF defined as left ventricular ejection fraction (LVEF) less than 40% and HFpEF defined as LVEF greater than 40%, 90-day mortality was 9.5% to 9.8% for both, and the risk of rehospitalization was 29.2% to 29.9%.[13]

While it is clear that both the high mortality and hospitalization rates associated with HF represent a global health problem, the relationship between hospitalizations and mortality is less clear. Patients are clearly at increased risk of death after an admission for HF, and this increased risk is directly related to the duration and frequency of HF hospitalizations.[16] However, it remains unknown whether reducing hospitalizations for HF will have a beneficial or adverse effect on mortality. An initial report based on the Medicare database demonstrated that an increased 30-day readmission rate from 17.2% to 20.1% was associated with decreased in-hospital (8.5%–4.3%) and 30-day mortality (12.8%–10.7%) during the period from 1993 to 2006.[9] Even when adjusted for multiple factors, comparison of Medicare hospital admission and mortality rates for HF demonstrated that mortality inversely correlated with hospital admission, although accounted for a relatively small portion of the overall estimates of variance.[22] A study from the Veterans Affairs system followed patients after their first admission for HF, and noted that mortality at 30 days decreased from 7.1% to 5.0%, whereas rehospitalizations during the same period actually increased from 5.6% to 6.1%.[23]

Causes of Mortality for HF Patients

Death in patients with diagnosed HF is most likely to be cardiovascular (CV) in nature (**Table 2**).[12,24–33] From a broad selection of HF trials with greater than 1000 patients, 78.0% to 96.2% of deaths were attributed to CV causes. The relative proportion adjudicated to circulatory failure or sudden cardiac death (SCD) differed by study, but constituted 26.1% to 47.8% and 22.7% to 50.9% of events, respectively. An analysis of 6 smaller heterogeneous trials with a total of 2014 combined deaths found similar results.[34] The frequency ranges for the less common CV causes of death were 1.6% to 7.0% for acute myocardial infarction (AMI), 1.6% to 5.1% for cerebrovascular accident (CVA), and less than 1% for pulmonary embolism.[12,13,29,30,32,33,35]

Few data exist on the type of decompensations that comprise those events labeled circulatory failure; however, they appear to contain both low cardiac output and congestive states. A Japanese registry of 323 post-hospitalization HF deaths broke down circulatory failure into primarily low output (13%), primarily congestion (14%), and the combination of low output with congestion (64%).[36] The underlying reasons for worsening HF likely include multiple external factors, although most have been studied only in terms of readmission (**Table 3**). However, biochemical changes such as progressive fibrosis or new myocyte dysfunction are not measured because tissue sampling is not part of routine clinical assessment.

Non-CV death contributes less to mortality than CV demise; however, the burden is substantial and ranges from 3.8% to 22.0% of HF patient deaths (see **Table 2**). The 2 principal causes of non-CV death are infection and neoplasm. In GISSI-HF, 12.0% of all deaths were due to neoplasms.[35] In CORONA, the 20.2% of non-CV deaths comprised 8.3% from infection, 6.9% from neoplasm, and less than 1% from gastrointestinal bleeding.[33] In the 23% of non-CV deaths in the 323 subjects in the Japanese registry, 37% were neoplastic, 27% infectious, 15% due to renal dysfunction, and 12% pulmonary.[36]

Causes of Readmission for HF Patients

Hospital diagnoses indicate that most HF patients are readmitted for CV reasons. HF is the most common individual cause but, in contrast to mortal events, a greater percentage of readmissions are non-CV (see **Table 1**; **Table 4**). From HF trials, previously hospitalized patients average 68.0% of readmissions from CV causes, 41.4% from worsening or exacerbated HF, and 32.0% from non-CV causes (see **Table 4**).[12,33,35,37–40] By comparison, HF patients who have not been previously hospitalized for HF have 16.5% of admissions attributable to worsening HF, 21.6% due to other CV conditions, and 61.9% resulting from non-CV causes.[41]

CV causes of readmission increase over time from discharge, and the majority of HF admissions occur in previously diagnosed HF patients. In an ADHERE analysis of previously hospitalized HF patients, 54.4% to 55.7% of readmissions were CV at 30 days, but 63.8% to 64.7% were CV at 1 year.[14] The proportion of non-CV admissions in Medicare patients with HF decreases over time after index admission (see **Table 1**).[14] Of patients admitted with HF, at least 75% are previously diagnosed HF, 20% de novo HF, and less

Table 2
Mode of death in select HF studies

Trial	No. of Subjects	CV Mortality (%)	Pump-Failure Mortality (%)	Sudden Cardiac Death (%)	CV Mortality (Other) (%)	Non-CV Mortality (%)	Authors,[Ref.] Year
SOLVD-T	2569	89.4	47.8	22.7	18.9	10.6	SOLVD Investigators,[24] 1991
SOLVD-P	4228	87.0	29.5	31.4	26.1	13.0	SOLVD Investigators,[25] 1992
ACE Overview	7105	85.2	44.2	27.7	13.3	14.8	Garg & Yusuf,[26] 1995
US Carvedilol	1094	96.2	34.0	50.9	11.3	3.8	Packer et al,[27] 1996
DIG	6800	85.1	35.5	40.1	9.5	14.9	[28]
PRAISE	1153	89.1	40.0	44.8	4.3	10.9	O'Connor et al,[29] 1998
ATLAS	3164	88.5	32.1	42.5	13.9	11.5	Poole-Wilson et al,[30] 2003
COMPANION	1520	78.0	44.4	26.5	7.1	22.0	Carson et al,[31] 2005
COMET	3029	87.4	32.8	43.1	11.5	12.6	Remme et al,[32] 2007
CORONA	5011	79.8	26.1	43.7	10.0	20.2	Kjekshus et al,[33] 2007
EVEREST	4133	86.8	47.2	30.0	9.6	13.2	O'Connor et al,[12] 2010
Total	39806						
Range	1153–7105	78.0–96.2	26.1–47.8	22.7–50.9	4.3–26.1	3.8–22.0	
Size-weighted average		85.7	37.2	35.6	12.9	14.3	

Data from O'Connor CM, Carson PE, Miller AB, et al. Effect of amlodipine on mode of death among patients with advanced heart failure in the PRAISE trial. Am J Cardiol 1998;82(7):881–7.

Table 3
Precipitating factors for admissions for HF

Trial	Total Admissions	Pulmonary Process or Infection (%)	Ischemia (%)	Arrhythmia (%)	Uncontrolled Hypertension (%)	Medication or Dietary Nonadherence (%)	Renal Dysfunction (%)	Other Identifiable Precipitant (%)	Unidentified (%)	Authors,[Ref.] Year
—	101	11.9	5.9	28.7	43.6	64.4	—	—	—	Ghali et al,[43] 1988
—	304	23.0	14.0	24.0	—	15.0	—	15.0	9.0	Opasich et al,[44] 1996
—	435	16.0	33.0	8.0	15.0	21.0	—	—	34.0	Chin et al,[45] 1997
—	179	—	13.4	6.1	5.6	41.9	—	18.4	14.5	Michalsen et al,[46] 1998
IN-CHF	215	12.0	5.0	5.0	5.0	21.0	—	17.0	40.0	Opasich et al,[47] 2001
NYHF Registry	619	8.0	10.0	9.0	13.0	12.8	9.5	13.9	—	Klapholz et al,[48] 2004
EHFS-II	3580	17.6	30.2	32.4	—	22.2	—	26.8	—	Nieminen et al,[18] 2006
—	428	29.0	10.0	21.9	13.3	18.5	—	28.3	—	Formiga et al,[49] 2007
OPTIMIZE-HF	48612	15.3	14.7	13.5	10.7	15.4	—	—	38.7	Fonarow et al,[50] 2008
GWTG-HF	54322	13.1	8.4	11.3	8.1	10.3	6.7	14.4	—	Ambardekar et al,[51] 2009
OFICA	1658	27.2	13.4	23.7	6.2	—	—	—	—	Logeart et al,[52] 2012
Total admissions	110453									
Range	101–54322	8.0–29.0	5.0–33.0	5.0–32.4	5.0–43.6	10.3–64.4				
Size-weighted average		14.5	12.1	13.2	9.0	13.0				

Note: multiple precipitants could be identified in the same patient.

Table 4
Cause of hospital admission in select HF studies

Trial	Total Readmissions	CV Readmission (%)	HF Readmission (%)	Non-CV Readmission (%)	Authors,[Ref.] Year
COPERNICUS	804	70.0	58.0	30.0	Packer et al,[37] 2002
CORONA	7768	61.2	31.0	38.8	Kjekshus et al,[33] 2007
GISSI-HF	2564	81.6	49.3	18.4	GISSI-HF Investigators,[35] 2008
HEAAL	2176	72.9	43.7	27.0	Konstam et al,[38] 2009
EVEREST	5239	60.8	46.5	39.2	O'Connor et al,[12] 2010
SHIFT	2587	81.1	45.8	18.9	Swedberg et al,[39] 2010
EMPHASIS-HF	899	78.2	46.4	21.8	Zannad et al,[40] 2011
Total readmissions	22037				
Range	804–7768	60.8–81.6	31.0–58.0	18.4–39.2	
Size-weighted average		68.0	41.4	32.0	
Registry					
ADHERE (30-d)	16518	55.6		44.4	Kociol et al,[14] 2010
Medicare (30-d)	123377	54.4		45.6	Kociol et al,[14] 2010
Medicare (30-d)	176125		37.0		Jencks et al,[1] 2009
ADHERE (1-y)	48802	64.6		35.3	Kociol et al,[14] 2010
Medicare (1-y)	349990	63.8		36.2	Kociol et al,[14] 2010

than 5% end-stage HF requiring advanced therapies.[10,42]

The 5 most commonly cited precipitating factors preceding HF admission are a pulmonary or infectious process (identified in 14.5% of HF exacerbations), cardiac arrhythmia (13.2%), medication or dietary nonadherence (13.0%), myocardial ischemia (12.1%), and uncontrolled hypertension (9.0%) (see **Table 3**).[18,43–52] In the cited investigations, more than 1 precipitant was involved in 19% of the subjects.[50] In one prospective study, HF exacerbations with or without resultant admission were also due to use of calcium-channel blockers (13%) and inappropriate physician changes in therapy (10%).[53]

Medication and dietary noncompliance are common and preventable causes of morbidity (see **Table 3**). In the HART trial, monitored electronic medication bottles detected a patient nonadherence rate of 37%.[54] Multiple factors cause medication noncompliance. In 183 patients followed over 3 years, 29% were at some point noncompliant. Of those, 50% had no medical justification, 30% stopped because of an adverse reaction, and 15% discontinued for some other medical reason.[55] Certain patients tend to be

very poorly compliant. In 202 patients followed for 6 months, 77.7% demonstrated 93% adherence, whereas 22.3% of patients showed initially poor 63.5% adherence which steeply declined to 39.1% during the study.[56]

The underlying causes of noncompliance are diverse, and include medication attributes such as dosing schedules as well as socioeconomic, educational, and social-status components.[57] Noncompliant patients tend to be younger, male, of minority race, lack insurance, and partake of more alcohol and tobacco. Income inequality is associated with noncompliance and readmission.[51,54,58–60] Medication adherence varies regionally and total per-person medication spending does not appear to correlate with level of adherence, but patients with prescription medication insurance are 26% to 32% more likely to fill their prescriptions.[60,61]

Improper physician-instituted therapy is also morbid, preventable, and common. Only 24.2% of IMPROVE-HF patients were taking all evidence-based modalities for which they were eligible.[62] Multiple registries demonstrate that only 60% to 80% of HFrEF patients are discharged on an angiotensin-converting enzyme (ACE) inhibitor, and 70% to 80% on a β-blocker.[13] In the HART trial only 63% of physicians followed clinical practice guidelines, and in only 41% of cases were both the physician and patient adherent to guideline-based therapies.[54] Many patients also do not have their HF medications increased to goal dosing.[63] Comorbidities specifically associated with suboptimal medication regimens include asthma and renal dysfunction, likely because of concerns for bronchospasm and worsening glomerular filtration with β-blockers and ACE inhibitors respectively.[54] Patients who are prescribed and titrate these evidence-based therapies have better outcomes in real-world observational analyses as well as in numerous controlled trials.[12,17]

Nonetheless, non-CV diseases cause 21% to 39% of HF patient readmissions.[1,50] The most common non-CV reasons for readmission are pulmonary processes including pneumonia and chronic obstructive pulmonary disease (COPD).[7] Specifically, pneumonia causes 5.1%, renal injury 3.9%, and nutritional or metabolic derangement 3.1% of Medicare readmissions.[1] In the OPTIMIZE-HF registry, 15.3% of admissions were pulmonary with 6.8% attributable to renal dysfunction.[50] Although part of the overlap in these admitting diagnoses may be due to true comorbidity, faulty diagnosis may also skew these data. Pneumonia and COPD exacerbations are difficult to distinguish from HF exacerbations, and emergency department diagnostic accuracy ranges from only 50% to 80%.[64,65]

MANAGEMENT GOALS
Therapeutic Targets

HF is a heterogeneous syndrome of congestion with or without decreased cardiac output that is common to varied underlying structural and functional etiology. Treatment goals and modalities differ between HF patients with distinct causes or at different points in progression.[66] Although HFpEF exists in half of HF patients and consists of diastolic dysfunction, the etiology is controversial and heterogeneous.[67] Abnormal relaxation may occur secondary to uncontrolled hypertension, as treatment of hypertension does prevent HFpEF as well as HFrEF; however, it may occur in other situations as well.[67,68] Because of a lack of understanding, therapeutic targets and evidence-based therapies are absent; therefore, HFpEF has a treatment paradigm that focuses on managing congestion and comorbidities.[69] By contrast, many complicated systemic interactions underlying HFrEF have been characterized, and multiple effective therapies have been delineated. Prevention of adverse events in HFrEF patients

requires reducing cardiac injury, inhibiting maladaptive systemic responses, and controlling relevant comorbidities. Many interventions that decrease mortality or hospital admission also improve quality of life.[66]

HFrEF is initiated by cardiac injury, often ischemia, with resultant neurohumoral induction of myocardial and extracellular matrix remodeling. The known activated signaling axes are primarily renin-angiotensin-aldosterone system and the sympathetic nervous system,[66] but multiple other pathways are undoubtedly involved. These changes lead to further reduced systolic function, ventricular dilation, and conduction abnormalities, including ventricular tachycardia. Maladaptive signaling and hemodynamic effects damage the myocardium, vasculature, kidneys, skeletal muscle, lungs, liver, and bone marrow.[70–72] These changes lead to acute HF (AHF) manifest by symptomatic vascular congestion that may be concomitant with low cardiac output. Recent data suggest that an AHF episode represents a complex, decompensated pathophysiologic state associated with significant end-organ damage. Increases in circulating troponin that indicate myocardial damage are common in AHF and portend a poor prognosis.[73,74] Similarly, worsening renal and other organ dysfunction is evident in patients with AHF, which are also linked to increased mortality.[75] This emerging paradigm of AHF as a period of end-organ damage supports a hypothesis that early treatment of the AHF event with agents that prevent or reduce such end-organ damage might also improve long-term outcomes.[76]

PHARMACOLOGIC STRATEGIES
Inpatient Pharmacologic Therapy

Overall poor inpatient quality of care and lack of guideline-based therapy is associated with higher readmission rates.[77] Patients with early decreased dyspnea or lower congestion scores at discharge have reduced organ damage, all-cause mortality, and readmission rates,[6,71,78,79] although 45% of patients are discharged with persistent congestion.[13] Patients with decreased markers of multiorgan damage also have improved outcomes.[70,75,76] Diuretics, vasodilators such as nitrates or nitroprusside, and various inotropes can decongest.

Loop diuretics typically initiate treatment, with subsequent addition of vasodilators, thiazide diuretics, and (rarely) inotropes if necessary. Therapies are titrated to clinical intravascular euvolemia, as use of a routine pulmonary artery catheter does not improve outcomes.[80,81] Bolus and infusion dosing of loop diuretics are equivalent; neither improve mortality, although higher doses induce greater volume loss.[82] Intravenous nitrates decrease myocardial ischemia and intubation rates in patients with pulmonary edema, but do not affect mortality.[83] Multiple other vasodilating therapies, including tezosentan, nesiritide, rolofylline, and tolvaptan, have failed to demonstrate beneficial effects on long-term outcomes.[84–87] The impotence of diuretics and vasodilators may be because they are relatively poor at reducing congestion. Twenty five percent of patients had no improvement and only 15% had complete resolution of congestion by 72 hours in DOSE, and just 10% of patients resolved venous congestion, edema, and orthopnea by 96 hours in CARRESS-HF.[82,88] Only the combination of vasodilators and diuretics reduced in-hospital mortality in the ALARM-HF registry, and the combination of isosorbide dinitrate with hydralazine decreased readmissions and mortality solely in self-described African Americans.[89,90]

The unproductive results with decongestive therapies may alternatively stem from intrinsic negative effects on neurohumoral signaling, direct organ toxicity, or counterproductive hemodynamic changes. Vasodilators increase hypotension and, although nitroprusside may improve decongestion and mortality, it has not been studied in a randomized prospective trial.[91] Vasopressor therapy consistently increases inpatient and outpatient mortality.[90] Fewer than 10% of admitted HF patients receive inotropic support, but these medications increase arrhythmias as well as hypotension, and their routine use worsens prognosis.[92–95]

Uniquely among AHF vasoactive therapies, serelaxin has shown promise in improving outcomes in patients admitted for AHF. In the 234-patient, dose-finding Pre-RELAX-AHF study, serelaxin (30 μg/kg/d) was associated with trends toward improved signs and symptoms of HF and reductions in worsening of HF, as well as improved survival, albeit based on very small numbers of events.[96] RELAX-AHF was an international, multicenter, randomized, placebo-controlled, phase III trial in 1161 patients, in which serelaxin treatment resulted in significant improvements in dyspnea and other signs and symptoms of HF, fewer events with worsening of HF, reduced duration of care in the intensive care unit/cardiac care unit and length of index hospital stay, and decreased markers of organ injury, all of which were associated with improved survival.[75,76] Whereas few have questioned the plausibility of a 48-hour infusion of milrinone, a therapy that can cause initial myocyte necrosis, to have a negative effect on long-term outcomes,[92] some have challenged the plausibility of serelaxin, a therapy that reduces initial end-organ damage, to have a beneficial long-term survival benefit.

Once the patient is stabilized, the priority should transition to initiation of chronic medical therapy. Modalities initiated in the hospital engender increased outpatient adherence and improved outcomes.[97] β-Blockers, ACE inhibitors, or angiotensin receptor blockers (ARBs), and mineralocorticoid receptor antagonists (MRAs) all should be started before discharge.[17,97–99] The patient should also be started on chronic therapy for their relevant comorbidities, particularly those that cause readmission such as pulmonary disease, vascular disease, and hypertension (see **Table 3**). Evidence and guideline-based therapies for these problems should be used.[100–105]

Outpatient Pharmacologic Therapy

A focal element of outpatient HF treatment is continued guideline-based medical and device therapy. Much of these data are for HFrEF and have been extensively reviewed in HF guidelines.[24,28,37,40,66,89,106–121] β-Blockade decreases mortality and readmissions with HFrEF,[27,109,110] and may correlate with declines in both with HFpEF.[13,122] ACE inhibitors (and ARBs) decrease mortality and readmissions with HFrEF and probably with HFpEF.[24,107,123–125] MRAs decrease mortality and readmissions with HFrEF.[112,126] Cardiac resynchronization therapy in appropriate patients decreases mortality and readmissions with HFrEF,[127] as does implantation of a cardioverter-defibrillator.[116,128] Digoxin decreases readmissions with HFrEF without a mortality benefit, and should be considered only after those therapies that decrease patient mortality.[28] For all these medications except digoxin, physicians should try to reach the highest possible doses tolerated, consistent with doses used in the major trials.[66] Long-term outcomes with diuretic therapy have not been studied, although they should continue to be used to relieve symptoms and signs of congestion.[66,78]

Many potential medical strategies have demonstrated no benefit or harm in HF patients. Although 57% to 62% of HF patients have a history of coronary artery disease and deserve aspirin therapy, trial data are lacking for HF patients without known ischemic disease.[14,42,129–131] A meta-analysis of 4 randomized controlled trials of warfarin for HF without other indications demonstrated no decrease in mortality, no decrease in AMI, and no decrease in admissions.[132] Warfarin did decrease CVAs in HFrEF when compared with aspirin, but with increased bleeding.[129] Ivabradine decreased mortality and readmission with HFrEF; however, most patients randomized were not on appropriately dosed β-blockade.[39,133] Rosuvastatin decreased HF patient readmission but not mortality in one trial but not in another, and should be used only in patients with other indications.[33,35] Amiodarone for arrhythmia prevention has a neutral to negative effect.[116,134] Although 74% of HF patients have hypertension[14] and uncontrolled hypertension is a frequent cause of readmission, amlodipine increased admissions for pulmonary edema in PRAISE.[135]

Pharmacologic Therapy for Comorbidities

One-half to two-thirds of admissions and mortality in previously hospitalized HF patients are not due to HF. Hypertension, ischemic disease, and arrhythmias are the most common culprit non-HF CV diseases (see **Tables 2** and **3**), although diabetes mellitus (DM), anemia, peripheral vascular, and renal disease are associated with adverse outcomes.[6] HFrEF is associated with higher rates of coronary artery disease, DM, hyperlipidemia, and tobacco smoking, whereas HFpEF is more strongly associated with hypertension, atrial fibrillation, COPD, and anemia.[20] Treatment of these comorbidities should follow guideline-based therapy, including the avoidance of calcium-channel blockade with HFrEF.[66,100–105] Patients should be evaluated for oral anticoagulation to treat atrial fibrillation, present in 31% to 37% of HF patients in the ADHERE registry. Although HFpEF patients have a higher incidence of atrial fibrillation, they are less likely to be initiated on warfarin.[13,14,42,66] Thirty-seven percent of all admitted HF patients deserve statin therapy for hyperlipidemia.[14] DM exists in 43% to 44% of hospitalized HF patients,[17,42,50] and should be treated with guideline-based therapy while avoiding thiazolidinediones that can provoke HF.[66,104]

COPD is present in 27.6% to 31% of hospitalized HF patients,[42,50] with HFpEF patients less likely than HFrEF patients to be counseled to quit smoking.[13] Physicians should vaccinate HF patients against influenza and pneumococcus, and use additional guideline-based treatment for COPD.[105] HF patients with COPD are less likely to receive all evidence-based therapies, specifically ACE inhibitors and β-blockers, perhaps because of concern for impairment of bronchodilation with concomitant β-blockade and cough with ACE inhibition.[54,136] However, a recent retrospective analysis of hospitalized COPD exacerbations demonstrated no worsening mortality or hospitalization with β-blockers, even in acute COPD exacerbations.[137] Based on this evidence, β-blockers appear to be safe in at least mild to moderate COPD. Nonetheless, as pulmonary causes are the second most common precipitating factor in HF readmission, use of β-blockade in COPD patients with HF deserves a randomized controlled trial.[1,50]

Chronic kidney disease (CKD) is present in 19.6% to 30% of hospitalized HF patients and predicts adverse events.[6,42,50] Acute kidney injury (AKI) and electrolyte abnormalities are associated with multiple HF therapies including diuretics, ACE inhibitors, and MRAs. CKD with HF is challenging because of the competing need for continued adequate glomerular filtration, maximal medical therapy, and medication toxicity. Although only 5% of hospitalized HF patients require dialysis, AKI is the cause of admission in 3.1% of Medicare patients and 6.7% to 9.5% of HF trial patients.[1,42] Attention to nephrology guidelines and consultation is prudent, with routine laboratory evaluation for worsening renal function and electrolyte derangements as well as avoidance of nephrotoxic medications such as nonsteroidal anti-inflammatories.[138,139]

The 2 most common mortal non-CV HF comorbidities are infection and neoplasia. Although most infections are not truly preventable, several common infections can be limited. Regional guidelines for adult vaccination should be followed including those against pneumococcus, tetanus, pertussis, influenza, herpes zoster, and others.[140] Cancer is the third most common cause of mortality in HF patients, so practitioners should remain vigilant using evidence-based cancer screening strategies consistent with regional and national guidelines.[141]

Patients with mental illness, specifically depression, frequently have worse outcomes than similar patients without the diagnosis. In the ADHERE registry, 10.6% of patients had a history of depression, and those patients had increased mortality at 6 to 9 months' follow-up.[142] A meta-analysis of HF patients reported depression in 21.5% with a range of 9% to 60%, associated with medication noncompliance.[55,143] Unfortunately, there are only a few small therapeutic trials for HF-associated depression, and no robust benefits have been demonstrated.[143]

NONPHARMACOLOGIC STRATEGIES
Inpatient Nonpharmacologic Therapy

Interventions other than medication and implantable-device therapy are also warranted in admitted HF patients, although the evidence is less robust. There is no evidence supporting oxygen therapy in HF patients who are not hypoxic, as data suggest that it may be detrimental.[70,144]

However, noninvasive positive pressure ventilation (NIPPV) improves hemodynamics, symptoms, and metabolic abnormalities,[145] and may reduce intubation and hospital mortality in patients with pulmonary edema.[146] An early study of ultrafiltration in patients admitted for AHF demonstrated greater weight loss with no difference in dyspnea at 48 hours in comparison with a diuretic, as well as the intriguing, hypothesis-generating finding of a reduction in unplanned or urgent clinical care or rehospitalizations for HF after discharge.[147] In the 188-patient CARRESS-HF study, ultrafiltration worsened renal dysfunction in comparison with diuretics in a different patient population with AHF and cardiorenal syndrome.[88]

Deconditioning, poor nutrition, and a decline in independent mobility are common. A meta-analysis of 22 studies of exercise training in either inpatient or outpatient settings demonstrated no change in adverse events, although overall the patients did show improvement in exercise capacity, 6-minute walk distance, and quality of life.[148] The duration of these studies (<1 year) may have underpowered them to detect any effect on outcomes, whereas a small study of 123 patients exercising twice weekly over 10 years demonstrated both decreased hospital admission and mortality.[120] Although lower albumin levels in discharged patients predict readmission, there has been no therapeutic trial of nutrition therapy in this population.[149,150]

In the current system of rapid hospital discharges, it is unclear whether hospital length of stay (LOS) correlates with overall HF outcomes. The average LOS for index HF admissions is 4 to 6 days in the United States, although readmission stays are 0.6 days longer. LOS can be significantly greater in other countries.[10,13,16,18,42,50,52] In the Veterans Affairs system, patient LOS decreased from 5.44 to 3.98 days between 1997 to 2010 as 30-day readmission rates declined from 16.5% to 13.8%, and 30-day mortality from 6.4% to 4.8%.[151] Nevertheless, hospitals with LOS significantly less than the mean had increased readmission rates. Medicare patient LOS also decreased from 8.8 days to 6.3 days between 1993 and 2006, with decreased in-hospital (8.5%–4.3%) and 30-day mortality (12.8%–10.7%). However, 30-day readmission increased from 17.2% to 20.1% and 30-day postdischarge mortality increased by 2.1%.[9]

Outpatient Nonpharmacologic Therapy

Care planning, patient education, and scheduled follow-up do prevent readmission, but location of discharge does not. Increased utilization of skilled nursing facilities does not correlate with 30-day readmission in HF patients.[152] However, clinical follow-up within 7 days of discharge is associated with reduced admission.[153] HF therapy is multifaceted and complicated, but only 54% to 66% of HF patients in OPTIMIZE-HF[17] and 32.3% of patients in ADHERE were given full discharge including medication management and follow-up.[42]

Education improves HF care.[51] A systematic review demonstrated that reduced prescription medication copayments, case management, patient education, and behavioral support all improve overall medication compliance.[154] Furthermore, multiple studies have shown 35% to 41% decreased rehospitalization or death with education, with smaller benefits from reminder phone calls and pharmacist-based interventions.[154–156] Comprehensive discharge planning consisting of medication counseling, follow-up home visits, patient education, and dietary and social services counseling also reduce readmission, with a relative risk of 0.75 and a number needed to treat of 12.[115]

Dietary and nutritional management are common aspects of HF therapy, although supportive data are lacking. A meta-analysis of sodium restriction in 6 randomized controlled trials of 2747 patients with HFrEF demonstrated worse outcomes. Specifically, a low-sodium diet of less than 2 g daily compared with 2 to 3 g daily increased mortality by increasing HF, SCD, and rehospitalization. The number needed to harm for any adverse outcome was 8.[157] A single-center underpowered randomized controlled trial demonstrated that a 1-L daily fluid restriction improved quality of life without changes in 60-day hospitalization or mortality. However, only 60% of patients were adherent with the restriction.[158] Lower caloric intake and body mass do predict adverse outcomes.[122] Lower outpatient albumin levels and nutrition scores correlate with increased probability of readmission, but there is no prospective intervention that has improved morbidity or mortality.[149,150] There is no evidence for benefit in any CV outcome by vitamin supplementation.[159]

Coordination of Care

Comorbidities and nonclinical attributes of all HF patients may be best treated by multidisciplinary interventions that address medical, psychosocial, behavioral, and socioeconomic issues.[160] A Cochrane review of 25 trials with at least 6 months of follow-up concurs.[121] Case management with telephone calls and home visits by specialist nurses decreases all-cause mortality at 12 months by 34% with no decrease in HF or CV mortality.[121,161] This approach and long-term exercise training are the few nonpharmacologic interventions that reduce mortality to a level comparable with that of medical and device therapies. Part of this improvement may be due to increased medication adherence.[154] Case management also decreases HF readmission by around 25% at 6 and 12 months. Multidisciplinary team-based care in and of itself also appears to have merit. A meta-analysis that excluded trials focusing on education or telemedicine indicated that team-based holistic care after discharge had no effect on mortality but did decrease all-cause and HF readmission.[121] The ability of team-based care to address and improve the multiple causes of patient decompensation may explain the surprisingly small effect for attending specialty HF clinics, which typically consist of a single provider. HF specialty clinic follow-up demonstrates a nonsignificant decrease in all-cause mortality, all-cause readmission, and HF readmission.[121] Unfortunately, although most studies have demonstrated some benefit, implementation of multidisciplinary services is hampered by costs and limited health care resources.[162]

EVALUATION AND ADJUSTMENT
Monitoring and Titration of Therapy

Patients who are readmitted or die early after discharge appear to decline on a host of measures including vital signs, laboratory tests, and symptomatologic abnormalities.[163] There are an excess of these factors associated with poor outcomes in HF patients, but no cohesive prediction tool has been validated to use these data for therapeutic intervention.[122,160] Such a tool might risk-stratify patients to determine need for admission, and predict those that require more intensive therapy or longer hospitalizations. Possible tools have also performed poorly for general medicine, and C-statistics for readmission range between 0.6 and 0.7.[15,160]

HF patients discharged from hospital undergo a steep decline in monitoring, evaluation, and encouragement of appropriate therapy. Increased weight gain after hospital discharge (2 kg vs 1 kg) at 2 to 6 months is associated with elevated venous pressures and increased readmission.[164] In addition, 45% of patients with either HFpEF or HFrEF are discharged with persistent symptoms of congestion,[13] thus necessitating continued active diuresis. Weight gain precedes admission by at least 7 to 30 days,[78,161] which has led to the practice of home titration of diuretics to daily weights.[53] Unfortunately, patient-based diuretic titration at home does not show any benefit. In a systematic review of 9 studies there was a trend toward fewer admissions and deaths as well as increased quality of life, but most studies were statistically nonsignificant.[165]

Monitoring systems that rely less on patient input and decision making are therefore attractive. B-Type natriuretic peptide (BNP) is significantly elevated in acute decompensations of both HFrEF and HFpEF.[13] Evidence-based HF therapies decrease BNP levels.[12,63] A meta-analysis of 6 small randomized controlled trials of mostly HFrEF patients demonstrated a mortality advantage with a hazard ratio of 0.69 for BNP-guided therapy.[63] This improvement occurred without increased adverse effects, and was postulated to be secondary to increased use of evidence-based therapy. Because of study heterogeneity, readmissions were not included in the meta-analysis, but trended toward reduced hospitalization. The goal levels of BNP or NT-proBNP (amino-terminal pro-BNP) were typically less than 100 to 150 or 1000 to 2000 pg/mL, respectively.[166] Although the benefits seen in these trials may not be directly attributable to titration to an absolute BNP level, the resultant increased office visits and medication dosing did significantly improve outcomes.

Avoiding Admission

HF is second only to psychosis in acute-care use after hospital discharge.[8] However, it is likely that not all patients who present to the emergency department need to be readmitted.[167] In the ADHERE registry and in HF retrospective analyses, most patients were treated with only oral or intravenous diuretics. Only 3% of patients had admission systolic blood pressures lower than 90 mm Hg, 23% required mechanical ventilation, and 16% to 23% required other intravenous therapeutics.[53,95] There is currently no large randomized controlled trial to support not admitting patients with acute HF syndromes, but the continued high mortality rate after hospital admission argues for detrimental disease processes that are not necessarily resolved by admission.[42] It has been suggested that perhaps an HF observation unit will be developed to allow brief observation and help stem HF admissions.[167] Nevertheless, evidence-based emergency department prediction models are needed to classify HF patients to decrease hospital admissions and the cost burden on health care, while not unduly increasing their rate of other adverse outcomes.

SUMMARY

Hospitalized HF patients have poor outcomes. These patients primarily die from CV causes, with the origin being SCD and circulatory failure in 25% to 50% each. Non-CV causes of death are less common, and primarily attributable to infection and cancer. Readmission of HF patients is also often due to CV causes, with HF being the single largest, although a significant proportion is attributable to arrhythmias, cardiac ischemia, and uncontrolled hypertension. Non-CV causes for readmission make up one-third of readmissions, with primary causes being pulmonary disease and renal dysfunction. Many HF readmissions are complicated by medication or behavioral noncompliance. Prevention of adverse outcomes in hospitalized HF patients relies on preventing HF progression by initiating and titrating evidence-based therapy, ensuring continued adherence to that therapy, and preventing and treating comorbidities. Future trials are needed for interventions that address AHF, hospital LOS (early vs delayed discharge), HFpEF medical therapy, β-blockade in patients with COPD, prediction of adverse outcomes and hospital admission, nutritional therapy, cardiorenal syndrome, and home medication titration strategies.

REFERENCES

1. Jencks SF, Williams MV, Coleman EA. Rehospitalizations among patients in the Medicare fee-for-service program. N Engl J Med 2009;360(14):1418–28.
2. Krumholz HM. Post-hospital syndrome—an acquired, transient condition of generalized risk. N Engl J Med 2013;368(2):100–2.
3. Dharmarajan K, Hsieh AF, Lin Z, et al. Diagnoses and timing of 30-day readmissions after hospitalization for heart failure, acute myocardial infarction, or pneumonia. JAMA 2013;309(4):355–63.
4. Fang J, Mensah GA, Croft JB, et al. Heart failure-related hospitalization in the U.S., 1979 to 2004. J Am Coll Cardiol 2008;52(6):428–34.
5. Go AS, Mozaffarian D, Roger VL, et al. Heart disease and stroke statistics—2013 update: a report from the American Heart Association. Circulation 2013;127(1):e6–245.
6. Harjola VP, Follath F, Nieminen MS, et al. Characteristics, outcomes, and predictors of mortality at 3 months and 1 year in patients hospitalized for acute heart failure. Eur J Heart Fail 2010;12(3):239–48.
7. Aranda JM Jr, Johnson JW, Conti JB. Current trends in heart failure readmission rates: analysis of Medicare data. Clin Cardiol 2009;32(1):47–52.
8. Vashi AA, Fox JP, Carr BG, et al. Use of hospital-based acute care among patients recently discharged from the hospital. JAMA 2013;309(4):364–71.
9. Bueno H, Ross JS, Wang Y, et al. Trends in length of stay and short-term outcomes among Medicare patients hospitalized for heart failure, 1993-2006. JAMA 2010;303(21):2141–7.
10. Cole RT, Gheorghiade M, Georgiopoulou VV, et al. Reassessing the use of vasodilators in heart failure. Expert Rev Cardiovasc Ther 2012;10(9):1141–51.
11. Krumholz HM, Parent EM, Tu N, et al. Readmission after hospitalization for congestive heart failure among Medicare beneficiaries. Arch Intern Med 1997;157(1):99–104.
12. O'Connor CM, Miller AB, Blair JE, et al. Causes of death and rehospitalization in patients hospitalized with worsening heart failure and reduced left ventricular ejection fraction: results from Efficacy of Vasopressin Antagonism in Heart Failure Outcome Study with Tolvaptan (EVEREST) program. Am Heart J 2010;159(5):841–849.e841.
13. Fonarow GC, Stough WG, Abraham WT, et al. Characteristics, treatments, and outcomes of patients with preserved systolic function hospitalized for heart failure: a report from the OPTIMIZE-HF Registry. J Am Coll Cardiol 2007;50(8):768–77.
14. Kociol RD, Hammill BG, Fonarow GC, et al. Generalizability and longitudinal outcomes of a national heart failure clinical registry: comparison of Acute Decompensated Heart Failure National Registry (ADHERE) and non-ADHERE Medicare beneficiaries. Am Heart J 2010;160(5):885–92.
15. Kansagara D, Englander H, Salanitro A, et al. Risk prediction models for hospital readmission: a systematic review. JAMA 2011;306(15):1688–98.
16. Solomon SD, Dobson J, Pocock S, et al. Influence of nonfatal hospitalization for heart failure on subsequent mortality in patients with chronic heart failure. Circulation 2007;116(13):1482–7.
17. Fonarow GC, Abraham WT, Albert NM, et al. Association between performance measures and clinical outcomes for patients hospitalized with heart failure. JAMA 2007;297(1):61–70.
18. Nieminen MS, Brutsaert D, Dickstein K, et al. Euro-Heart Failure Survey II (EHFS II): a survey on hospitalized acute heart failure patients: description of population. Eur Heart J 2006;27(22):2725–36.
19. Blair JE, Zannad F, Konstam MA, et al. Continental differences in clinical characteristics, management, and outcomes in patients hospitalized with worsening heart failure results from the EVEREST (Efficacy of Vasopressin Antagonism in Heart Failure: Outcome Study with Tolvaptan) program. J Am Coll Cardiol 2008;52(20):1640–8.
20. Bhatia RS, Tu JV, Lee DS, et al. Outcome of heart failure with preserved ejection fraction in a population-based study. N Engl J Med 2006;355(3):260–9.
21. Ross JS, Normand SL, Wang Y, et al. Hospital volume and 30-day mortality for three common medical conditions. N Engl J Med 2010;362(12):1110–8.

22. Krumholz HM, Lin Z, Keenan PS, et al. Relationship between hospital readmission and mortality rates for patients hospitalized with acute myocardial infarction, heart failure, or pneumonia. JAMA 2013;309(6):587–93.

23. Heidenreich PA, Sahay A, Kapoor JR, et al. Divergent trends in survival and readmission following a hospitalization for heart failure in the Veterans Affairs health care system 2002 to 2006. J Am Coll Cardiol 2010;56(5):362–8.

24. Effect of enalapril on survival in patients with reduced left ventricular ejection fractions and congestive heart failure. The SOLVD Investigators. N Engl J Med 1991;325(5):293–302.

25. Effect of enalapril on mortality and the development of heart failure in asymptomatic patients with reduced left ventricular ejection fractions. The SOLVD Investigators. N Engl J Med 1992; 327(10):685–91.

26. Garg R, Yusuf S. Overview of randomized trials of angiotensin-converting enzyme inhibitors on mortality and morbidity in patients with heart failure. Collaborative Group on ACE Inhibitor Trials. JAMA 1995;273(18):1450–6.

27. Packer M, Bristow MR, Cohn JN, et al. The effect of carvedilol on morbidity and mortality in patients with chronic heart failure. U.S. Carvedilol Heart Failure Study Group. N Engl J Med 1996;334(21): 1349–55.

28. The effect of digoxin on mortality and morbidity in patients with heart failure. The Digitalis Investigation Group. N Engl J Med 1997;336(8):525–33.

29. O'Connor CM, Carson PE, Miller AB, et al. Effect of amlodipine on mode of death among patients with advanced heart failure in the PRAISE trial. Prospective Randomized Amlodipine Survival Evaluation. Am J Cardiol 1998;82(7):881–7.

30. Poole-Wilson PA, Uretsky BF, Thygesen K, et al. Mode of death in heart failure: findings from the ATLAS trial. Heart 2003;89(1):42–8.

31. Carson P, Anand I, O'Connor C, et al. Mode of death in advanced heart failure: the Comparison of Medical, Pacing, and Defibrillation Therapies in Heart Failure (COMPANION) trial. J Am Coll Cardiol 2005;46(12):2329–34.

32. Remme WJ, Cleland JG, Erhardt L, et al. Effect of carvedilol and metoprolol on the mode of death in patients with heart failure. Eur J Heart Fail 2007; 9(11):1128–35.

33. Kjekshus J, Apetrei E, Barrios V, et al. Rosuvastatin in older patients with systolic heart failure. N Engl J Med 2007;357(22):2248–61.

34. Mozaffarian D, Anker SD, Anand I, et al. Prediction of mode of death in heart failure: the Seattle Heart Failure Model. Circulation 2007;116(4):392–8.

35. Gissi HFI, Tavazzi L, Maggioni AP, et al. Effect of rosuvastatin in patients with chronic heart failure (the GISSI-HF trial): a randomised, double-blind, placebo-controlled trial. Lancet 2008;372(9645):1231–9.

36. Hamaguchi S, Kinugawa S, Sobirin MA, et al. Mode of death in patients with heart failure and reduced vs. preserved ejection fraction: report from registry of hospitalized heart failure patients. Circ J 2012; 76(7):1662–9.

37. Packer M, Fowler MB, Roecker EB, et al. Effect of carvedilol on the morbidity of patients with severe chronic heart failure: results of the carvedilol prospective randomized cumulative survival (COPERNICUS) study. Circulation 2002;106(17):2194–9.

38. Konstam MA, Neaton JD, Dickstein K, et al. Effects of high-dose versus low-dose losartan on clinical outcomes in patients with heart failure (HEAAL study): a randomised, double-blind trial. Lancet 2009;374(9704):1840–8.

39. Swedberg K, Komajda M, Bohm M, et al. Ivabradine and outcomes in chronic heart failure (SHIFT): a randomised placebo-controlled study. Lancet 2010;376(9744):875–85.

40. Zannad F, McMurray JJ, Krum H, et al. Eplerenone in patients with systolic heart failure and mild symptoms. N Engl J Med 2011;364(1):11–21.

41. Dunlay SM, Redfield MM, Weston SA, et al. Hospitalizations after heart failure diagnosis a community perspective. J Am Coll Cardiol 2009;54(18): 1695–702.

42. Adams KF Jr, Fonarow GC, Emerman CL, et al. Characteristics and outcomes of patients hospitalized for heart failure in the United States: rationale, design, and preliminary observations from the first 100,000 cases in the Acute Decompensated Heart Failure National Registry (ADHERE). Am Heart J 2005;149(2):209–16.

43. Ghali JK, Kadakia S, Cooper R, et al. Precipitating factors leading to decompensation of heart failure. Traits among urban blacks. Arch Intern Med 1988; 148(9):2013–6.

44. Opasich C, Febo O, Riccardi PG, et al. Concomitant factors of decompensation in chronic heart failure. Am J Cardiol 1996;78(3):354–7.

45. Chin MH, Goldman L. Factors contributing to the hospitalization of patients with congestive heart failure. Am J Public Health 1997;87(4):643–8.

46. Michalsen A, Konig G, Thimme W. Preventable causative factors leading to hospital admission with decompensated heart failure. Heart 1998; 80(5):437–41.

47. Opasich C, Rapezzi C, Lucci D, et al. Precipitating factors and decision-making processes of short-term worsening heart failure despite "optimal" treatment (from the IN-CHF Registry). Am J Cardiol 2001;88(4):382–7.

48. Klapholz M, Maurer M, Lowe AM, et al. Hospitalization for heart failure in the presence of a normal left ventricular ejection fraction: results of the New York

Heart Failure Registry. J Am Coll Cardiol 2004; 43(8):1432–8.

49. Formiga F, Chivite D, Manito N, et al. Hospitalization due to acute heart failure. Role of the precipitating factors. Int J Cardiol 2007;120(2):237–41.

50. Fonarow GC, Abraham WT, Albert NM, et al. Factors identified as precipitating hospital admissions for heart failure and clinical outcomes: findings from OPTIMIZE-HF. Arch Intern Med 2008;168(8): 847–54.

51. Ambardekar AV, Fonarow GC, Hernandez AF, et al. Characteristics and in-hospital outcomes for non-adherent patients with heart failure: findings from Get With The Guidelines—Heart Failure (GWTG-HF). Am Heart J 2009;158(4):644–52.

52. Logeart D, Isnard R, Resche-Rigon M, et al. Current aspects of the spectrum of acute heart failure syndromes in a real-life setting: the OFICA study. Eur J Heart Fail 2013;15(4):465–76.

53. Tsuyuki RT, McKelvie RS, Arnold JM, et al. Acute precipitants of congestive heart failure exacerbations. Arch Intern Med 2001;161(19):2337–42.

54. Calvin JE, Shanbhag S, Avery E, et al. Adherence to evidence-based guidelines for heart failure in physicians and their patients: lessons from the Heart Failure Adherence Retention Trial (HART). Congest Heart Fail 2012;18(2):73–8.

55. Mockler M, O'Loughlin C, Murphy N, et al. Causes and consequences of nonpersistence with heart failure medication. Am J Cardiol 2009;103(6):834–8.

56. Riegel B, Lee CS, Ratcliffe SJ, et al. Predictors of objectively measured medication nonadherence in adults with heart failure. Circ Heart Fail 2012; 5(4):430–6.

57. Wu JR, Moser DK, Chung ML, et al. Predictors of medication adherence using a multidimensional adherence model in patients with heart failure. J Card Fail 2008;14(7):603–14.

58. Wu JR, Moser DK, Chung ML, et al. Objectively measured, but not self-reported, medication adherence independently predicts event-free survival in patients with heart failure. J Card Fail 2008;14(3): 203–10.

59. Lindenauer PK, Lagu T, Rothberg MB, et al. Income inequality and 30 day outcomes after acute myocardial infarction, heart failure, and pneumonia: retrospective cohort study. BMJ 2013;346: f521.

60. DiMartino LD, Shea AM, Hernandez AF, et al. Use of guideline-recommended therapies for heart failure in the Medicare population. Clin Cardiol 2010; 33(7):400–5.

61. Zhang Y, Wu SH, Fendrick AM, et al. Variation in medication adherence in heart failure. JAMA Intern Med 2013;173(6):468–70.

62. Fonarow GC, Albert NM, Curtis AB, et al. Associations between outpatient heart failure process-of-care measures and mortality. Circulation 2011; 123(15):1601–10.

63. Felker GM, Hasselblad V, Hernandez AF, et al. Biomarker-guided therapy in chronic heart failure: a meta-analysis of randomized controlled trials. Am Heart J 2009;158(3):422–30.

64. Remes J, Miettinen H, Reunanen A, et al. Validity of clinical diagnosis of heart failure in primary health care. Eur Heart J 1991;12(3):315–21.

65. Di Bari M, Pozzi C, Cavallini MC, et al. The diagnosis of heart failure in the community. Comparative validation of four sets of criteria in unselected older adults: the ICARe Dicomano Study. J Am Coll Cardiol 2004;44(8):1601–8.

66. McMurray JJ, Adamopoulos S, Anker SD, et al. ESC guidelines for the diagnosis and treatment of acute and chronic heart failure 2012: the Task Force for the Diagnosis and Treatment of Acute and Chronic Heart Failure 2012 of the European Society of Cardiology. Developed in collaboration with the Heart Failure Association (HFA) of the ESC. Eur Heart J 2012;33(14):1787–847.

67. Oghlakian GO, Sipahi I, Fang JC. Treatment of heart failure with preserved ejection fraction: have we been pursuing the wrong paradigm? Mayo Clin Proc 2011;86(6):531–9.

68. Davis BR, Kostis JB, Simpson LM, et al. Heart failure with preserved and reduced left ventricular ejection fraction in the antihypertensive and lipid-lowering treatment to prevent heart attack trial. Circulation 2008;118(22):2259–67.

69. Borlaug BA, Paulus WJ. Heart failure with preserved ejection fraction: pathophysiology, diagnosis, and treatment. Eur Heart J 2011;32(6): 670–9.

70. Lee DS, Stitt A, Austin PC, et al. Prediction of heart failure mortality in emergent care: a cohort study. Ann Intern Med 2012;156(11):767–75, W-261, W-262.

71. Parrinello G, Di Pasquale P, Torres D, et al. Troponin I release after intravenous treatment with high furosemide doses plus hypertonic saline solution in decompensated heart failure trial (Tra-HSS-Fur). Am Heart J 2012;164(3):351–7.

72. Metra M, Cotter G, Gheorghiade M, et al. The role of the kidney in heart failure. Eur Heart J 2012; 33(17):2135–42.

73. O'Connor CM, Fiuzat M, Lombardi C, et al. Impact of serial troponin release on outcomes in patients with acute heart failure: analysis from the PROTECT pilot study. Circ Heart Fail 2011;4(6):724–32.

74. Peacock WF 4th, De Marco T, Fonarow GC, et al. Cardiac troponin and outcome in acute heart failure. N Engl J Med 2008;358(20):2117–26.

75. Metra M, Cotter G, Davison BA, et al. Effect of Serelaxin on Cardiac, Renal, and Hepatic Biomarkers in the Relaxin in Acute Heart Failure (RELAX-AHF)

development program: correlation with outcomes. J Am Coll Cardiol 2013;61(2):196–206.

76. Teerlink JR, Cotter G, Davison BA, et al. Serelaxin, recombinant human relaxin-2, for treatment of acute heart failure (RELAX-AHF): a randomised, placebo-controlled trial. Lancet 2013;381(9860): 29–39.

77. Ashton CM, Del Junco DJ, Souchek J, et al. The association between the quality of inpatient care and early readmission: a meta-analysis of the evidence. Med Care 1997;35(10):1044–59.

78. Ambrosy AP, Pang PS, Khan S, et al. Clinical course and predictive value of congestion during hospitalization in patients admitted for worsening signs and symptoms of heart failure with reduced ejection fraction: findings from the EVEREST trial. Eur Heart J 2013;34(11):835–43.

79. Mentz RJ, Hernandez AF, Stebbins A, et al. Predictors of early dyspnoea relief in acute heart failure and the association with 30-day outcomes: findings from ASCEND-HF. Eur J Heart Fail 2013; 15(4):456–64.

80. Binanay C, Califf RM, Hasselblad V, et al. Evaluation study of congestive heart failure and pulmonary artery catheterization effectiveness: the ESCAPE trial. JAMA 2005;294(13):1625–33.

81. Shah MR, Hasselblad V, Stevenson LW, et al. Impact of the pulmonary artery catheter in critically ill patients: meta-analysis of randomized clinical trials. JAMA 2005;294(13):1664–70.

82. Felker GM, Lee KL, Bull DA, et al. Diuretic strategies in patients with acute decompensated heart failure. N Engl J Med 2011;364(9):797–805.

83. Vizzardi E, Bonadei I, Rovetta R, et al. When should we use nitrates in congestive heart failure? Cardiovasc Ther 2013;31(1):27–31.

84. Konstam MA, Gheorghiade M, Burnett JC Jr, et al. Effects of oral tolvaptan in patients hospitalized for worsening heart failure: the EVEREST Outcome Trial. JAMA 2007;297(12):1319–31.

85. Massie BM, O'Connor CM, Metra M, et al. Rolofylline, an adenosine A1-receptor antagonist, in acute heart failure. N Engl J Med 2010;363(15):1419–28.

86. McMurray JJ, Teerlink JR, Cotter G, et al. Effects of tezosentan on symptoms and clinical outcomes in patients with acute heart failure: the VERITAS randomized controlled trials. JAMA 2007;298(17): 2009–19.

87. O'Connor CM, Starling RC, Hernandez AF, et al. Effect of nesiritide in patients with acute decompensated heart failure. N Engl J Med 2011; 365(1):32–43.

88. Bart BA, Goldsmith SR, Lee KL, et al. Ultrafiltration in decompensated heart failure with cardiorenal syndrome. N Engl J Med 2012;367(24):2296–304.

89. Taylor AL, Ziesche S, Yancy C, et al. Combination of isosorbide dinitrate and hydralazine in blacks with heart failure. N Engl J Med 2004;351(20): 2049–57.

90. Mebazaa A, Parissis J, Porcher R, et al. Short-term survival by treatment among patients hospitalized with acute heart failure: the global ALARM-HF registry using propensity scoring methods. Intensive Care Med 2011;37(2):290–301.

91. Mullens W, Abrahams Z, Francis GS, et al. Sodium nitroprusside for advanced low-output heart failure. J Am Coll Cardiol 2008;52(3):200–7.

92. Cuffe MS, Califf RM, Adams KF Jr, et al. Short-term intravenous milrinone for acute exacerbation of chronic heart failure: a randomized controlled trial. JAMA 2002;287(12):1541–7.

93. Mebazaa A, Nieminen MS, Packer M, et al. Levosimendan vs dobutamine for patients with acute decompensated heart failure: the SURVIVE randomized trial. JAMA 2007;297(17):1883–91.

94. Tacon CL, McCaffrey J, Delaney A. Dobutamine for patients with severe heart failure: a systematic review and meta-analysis of randomised controlled trials. Intensive Care Med 2012;38(3):359–67.

95. Abraham WT, Adams KF, Fonarow GC, et al. In-hospital mortality in patients with acute decompensated heart failure requiring intravenous vasoactive medications: an analysis from the Acute Decompensated Heart Failure National Registry (ADHERE). J Am Coll Cardiol 2005;46(1):57–64.

96. Teerlink JR, Metra M, Felker GM, et al. Relaxin for the treatment of patients with acute heart failure (Pre-RELAX-AHF): a multicentre, randomised, placebo-controlled, parallel-group, dose-finding phase IIb study. Lancet 2009;373:1429–39.

97. Fonarow GC, Abraham WT, Albert NM, et al. Carvedilol use at discharge in patients hospitalized for heart failure is associated with improved survival: an analysis from Organized Program to Initiate Lifesaving Treatment in Hospitalized Patients with Heart Failure (OPTIMIZE-HF). Am Heart J 2007; 153(1):82.e1–11.

98. Gattis WA, O'Connor CM, Gallup DS, et al. Predischarge initiation of carvedilol in patients hospitalized for decompensated heart failure: results of the Initiation Management Predischarge: process for Assessment of Carvedilol Therapy in Heart Failure (IMPACT-HF) trial. J Am Coll Cardiol 2004; 43(9):1534–41.

99. Bohm M, Link A, Cai D, et al. Beneficial association of beta-blocker therapy on recovery from severe acute heart failure treatment: data from the Survival of Patients With Acute Heart Failure in Need of Intravenous Inotropic Support trial. Crit Care Med 2011;39(5):940–4.

100. Tracy CM, Epstein AE, Darbar D, et al. 2012 ACCF/AHA/HRS focused update incorporated into the ACCF/AHA/HRS 2008 guidelines for device-based therapy of cardiac rhythm abnormalities: a

report of the American College of Cardiology Foundation/American Heart Association Task Force on Practice Guidelines and the Heart Rhythm Society. J Am Coll Cardiol 2013;61(3):e6–75.

101. Smith SC Jr, Benjamin EJ, Bonow RO, et al. AHA/ACCF secondary prevention and risk reduction therapy for patients with coronary and other atherosclerotic vascular disease: 2011 update: a guideline from the American Heart Association and American College of Cardiology Foundation. Circulation 2011;124(22):2458–73.

102. Fuster V, Ryden LE, Cannom DS, et al. 2011 ACCF/AHA/HRS focused updates incorporated into the ACC/AHA/ESC 2006 guidelines for the management of patients with atrial fibrillation: a report of the American College of Cardiology Foundation/American Heart Association Task Force on practice guidelines. Circulation 2011;123(10):e269–367.

103. Zipes DP, Camm AJ, Borggrefe M, et al. ACC/AHA/ESC 2006 guidelines for management of patients with ventricular arrhythmias and the prevention of sudden cardiac death: a report of the American College of Cardiology/American Heart Association Task Force and the European Society of Cardiology Committee for Practice Guidelines (Writing Committee to Develop Guidelines for Management of Patients With Ventricular Arrhythmias and the Prevention of Sudden Cardiac Death): developed in collaboration with the European Heart Rhythm Association and the Heart Rhythm Society. Circulation 2006;114(10):e385–484.

104. American Diabetes Association. Standards of medical care in diabetes—2013. Diabetes Care 2013;36(Suppl 1):S11–66.

105. Qaseem A, Wilt TJ, Weinberger SE, et al. Diagnosis and management of stable chronic obstructive pulmonary disease: a clinical practice guideline update from the American College of Physicians, American College of Chest Physicians, American Thoracic Society, and European Respiratory Society. Ann Intern Med 2011;155(3):179–91.

106. Cohn JN, Archibald DG, Ziesche S, et al. Effect of vasodilator therapy on mortality in chronic congestive heart failure. Results of a Veterans Administration Cooperative Study. N Engl J Med 1986;314(24):1547–52.

107. Effects of enalapril on mortality in severe congestive heart failure. Results of the Cooperative North Scandinavian Enalapril Survival Study (CONSENSUS). The CONSENSUS Trial Study Group. N Engl J Med 1987;316(23):1429–35.

108. Packer M, Poole-Wilson PA, Armstrong PW, et al. Comparative effects of low and high doses of the angiotensin-converting enzyme inhibitor, lisinopril, on morbidity and mortality in chronic heart failure. ATLAS Study Group. Circulation 1999;100(23):2312–8.

109. The Cardiac Insufficiency Bisoprolol Study II (CIBIS-II): a randomised trial. Lancet 1999;353(9146):9–13.

110. Effect of metoprolol CR/XL in chronic heart failure: Metoprolol CR/XL Randomised Intervention Trial in Congestive Heart Failure (MERIT-HF). Lancet 1999;353(9169):2001–7.

111. Hjalmarson A, Goldstein S, Fagerberg B, et al. Effects of controlled-release metoprolol on total mortality, hospitalizations, and well-being in patients with heart failure: the Metoprolol CR/XL Randomized Intervention Trial in congestive heart failure (MERIT-HF). MERIT-HF Study Group. JAMA 2000;283(10):1295–302.

112. Pitt B, Zannad F, Remme WJ, et al. The effect of spironolactone on morbidity and mortality in patients with severe heart failure. Randomized Aldactone Evaluation Study Investigators. N Engl J Med 1999;341(10):709–17.

113. Packer M, Coats AJ, Fowler MB, et al. Effect of carvedilol on survival in severe chronic heart failure. N Engl J Med 2001;344(22):1651–8.

114. Bristow MR, Saxon LA, Boehmer J, et al. Cardiac-resynchronization therapy with or without an implantable defibrillator in advanced chronic heart failure. N Engl J Med 2004;350(21):2140–50.

115. Phillips CO, Wright SM, Kern DE, et al. Comprehensive discharge planning with postdischarge support for older patients with congestive heart failure: a meta-analysis. JAMA 2004;291(11):1358–67.

116. Bardy GH, Lee KL, Mark DB, et al. Amiodarone or an implantable cardioverter-defibrillator for congestive heart failure. N Engl J Med 2005;352(3):225–37.

117. Cleland JG, Daubert JC, Erdmann E, et al. The effect of cardiac resynchronization on morbidity and mortality in heart failure. N Engl J Med 2005;352(15):1539–49.

118. O'Connor CM, Whellan DJ, Lee KL, et al. Efficacy and safety of exercise training in patients with chronic heart failure: HF-ACTION randomized controlled trial. JAMA 2009;301(14):1439–50.

119. Tang AS, Wells GA, Talajic M, et al. Cardiac-resynchronization therapy for mild-to-moderate heart failure. N Engl J Med 2010;363(25):2385–95.

120. Belardinelli R, Georgiou D, Cianci G, et al. 10-year exercise training in chronic heart failure: a randomized controlled trial. J Am Coll Cardiol 2012;60(16):1521–8.

121. Takeda A, Taylor SJ, Taylor RS, et al. Clinical service organisation for heart failure. Cochrane Database Syst Rev 2012;(9):CD002752.

122. Pocock SJ, Ariti CA, McMurray JJ, et al. Predicting survival in heart failure: a risk score based on 39 372 patients from 30 studies. Eur Heart J 2012;34(19):1404–13.

123. Cohn JN, Johnson G, Ziesche S, et al. A comparison of enalapril with hydralazine-isosorbide dinitrate in

the treatment of chronic congestive heart failure. N Engl J Med 1991;325(5):303–10.

124. Lund LH, Benson L, Dahlstrom U, et al. Association between use of renin-angiotensin system antagonists and mortality in patients with heart failure and preserved ejection fraction. JAMA 2012; 308(20):2108–17.

125. Yusuf S, Pfeffer MA, Swedberg K, et al. Effects of candesartan in patients with chronic heart failure and preserved left-ventricular ejection fraction: the CHARM-Preserved Trial. Lancet 2003; 362(9386):777–81.

126. Pitt B, Williams G, Remme W, et al. The EPHESUS trial: eplerenone in patients with heart failure due to systolic dysfunction complicating acute myocardial infarction. Eplerenone Post-AMI Heart Failure Efficacy and Survival Study. Cardiovasc Drugs Ther 2001;15(1):79–87.

127. McAlister FA, Ezekowitz JA, Wiebe N, et al. Systematic review: cardiac resynchronization in patients with symptomatic heart failure. Ann Intern Med 2004;141(5):381–90.

128. Moss AJ, Zareba W, Hall WJ, et al. Prophylactic implantation of a defibrillator in patients with myocardial infarction and reduced ejection fraction. N Engl J Med 2002;346(12):877–83.

129. Homma S, Thompson JL, Pullicino PM, et al. Warfarin and aspirin in patients with heart failure and sinus rhythm. N Engl J Med 2012;366(20): 1859–69.

130. Cleland JG, Findlay I, Jafri S, et al. The Warfarin/Aspirin Study in Heart failure (WASH): a randomized trial comparing antithrombotic strategies for patients with heart failure. Am Heart J 2004; 148(1):157–64.

131. Massie BM, Collins JF, Ammon SE, et al. Randomized trial of warfarin, aspirin, and clopidogrel in patients with chronic heart failure: the Warfarin and Antiplatelet Therapy in Chronic Heart Failure (WATCH) trial. Circulation 2009;119(12): 1616–24.

132. Rengo G, Pagano G, Squizzato A, et al. Oral anticoagulation therapy in heart failure patients in sinus rhythm: a systematic review and meta-analysis. PLoS One 2013;8(1):e52952.

133. Teerlink JR. Ivabradine in heart failure—no paradigm SHIFT…Yet. Lancet 2010;376(9744):847–9.

134. Singh SN, Fletcher RD, Fisher SG, et al. Amiodarone in patients with congestive heart failure and asymptomatic ventricular arrhythmia. Survival Trial of Antiarrhythmic Therapy in Congestive Heart Failure. N Engl J Med 1995;333(2):77–82.

135. Packer M, O'Connor CM, Ghali JK, et al. Effect of amlodipine on morbidity and mortality in severe chronic heart failure. Prospective Randomized Amlodipine Survival Evaluation Study Group. N Engl J Med 1996;335(15):1107–14.

136. Mentz RJ, Schmidt PH, Kwasny MJ, et al. The impact of chronic obstructive pulmonary disease in patients hospitalized for worsening heart failure with reduced ejection fraction: an analysis of the EVEREST Trial. J Card Fail 2012;18(7):515–23.

137. Stefan MS, Rothberg MB, Priya A, et al. Association between beta-blocker therapy and outcomes in patients hospitalised with acute exacerbations of chronic obstructive lung disease with underlying ischaemic heart disease, heart failure or hypertension. Thorax 2012;67(11):977–84.

138. Levey AS, Coresh J, Balk E, et al. National Kidney Foundation practice guidelines for chronic kidney disease: evaluation, classification, and stratification. Ann Intern Med 2003;139(2):137–47.

139. Khwaja A. KDIGO Clinical Practice Guidelines for Acute Kidney Injury. Nephron Clin Pract 2012; 120(4):179–84.

140. Advisory Committee on Immunization Practices. Recommended adult immunization schedule: United States, 2013. Ann Intern Med 2013;158(3): 191–9.

141. US Preventive Services Task Force. Screening for breast cancer: U.S. Preventive Services Task Force recommendation statement. Ann Intern Med 2009; 151(10):716–26.

142. Albert NM, Fonarow GC, Abraham WT, et al. Depression and clinical outcomes in heart failure: an OPTIMIZE-HF analysis. Am J Med 2009; 122(4):366–73.

143. Rutledge T, Reis VA, Linke SE, et al. Depression in heart failure: a meta-analytic review of prevalence, intervention effects, and associations with clinical outcomes. J Am Coll Cardiol 2006;48(8): 1527–37.

144. Park JH, Balmain S, Berry C, et al. Potentially detrimental cardiovascular effects of oxygen in patients with chronic left ventricular systolic dysfunction. Heart 2010;96(7):533–8.

145. Gray A, Goodacre S, Newby DE, et al. Noninvasive ventilation in acute cardiogenic pulmonary edema. N Engl J Med 2008;359(2):142–51.

146. Vital FM, Saconato H, Ladeira MT, et al. Non-invasive positive pressure ventilation (CPAP or bilevel NPPV) for cardiogenic pulmonary edema. Cochrane Database Syst Rev 2008;(3):CD005351.

147. Costanzo MR, Guglin ME, Saltzberg MT, et al. Ultrafiltration versus intravenous diuretics for patients hospitalized for acute decompensated heart failure. J Am Coll Cardiol 2007;49(6):675–83.

148. van der Meer S, Zwerink M, van Brussel M, et al. Effect of outpatient exercise training programmes in patients with chronic heart failure: a systematic review. Eur J Cardiovasc Prev Rehabil 2012;19(4): 795–803.

149. Kinugasa Y, Kato M, Sugihara S, et al. Geriatric nutritional risk index predicts functional

dependency and mortality in patients with heart failure with preserved ejection fraction. Circ J 2013;77(3):705–11.

150. Friedmann JM, Jensen GL, Smiciklas-Wright H, et al. Predicting early nonelective hospital readmission in nutritionally compromised older adults. Am J Clin Nutr 1997;65(6):1714–20.

151. Kaboli PJ, Go JT, Hockenberry J, et al. Associations between reduced hospital length of stay and 30-day readmission rate and mortality: 14-year experience in 129 Veterans Affairs hospitals. Ann Intern Med 2012;157(12):837–45.

152. Chen J, Ross JS, Carlson MD, et al. Skilled nursing facility referral and hospital readmission rates after heart failure or myocardial infarction. Am J Med 2012;125:100.e1–9.

153. Hernandez AF, Greiner MA, Fonarow GC, et al. Relationship between early physician follow-up and 30-day readmission among Medicare beneficiaries hospitalized for heart failure. JAMA 2010; 303(17):1716–22.

154. Viswanathan M, Golin CE, Jones CD, et al. Interventions to improve adherence to self-administered medications for chronic diseases in the United States: a systematic review. Ann Intern Med 2012;157(11):785–95.

155. Koelling TM, Johnson ML, Cody RJ, et al. Discharge education improves clinical outcomes in patients with chronic heart failure. Circulation 2005;111(2):179–85.

156. Juilliere Y, Jourdain P, Suty-Selton C, et al. Therapeutic patient education and all-cause mortality in patients with chronic heart failure: a propensity analysis. Int J Cardiol 2012. [Epub ahead of print].

157. Dinicolantonio JJ, Pasquale PD, Taylor RS, et al. Low sodium versus normal sodium diets in systolic heart failure: systematic review and meta-analysis. Heart 2013. [Epub ahead of print].

158. Albert NM, Nutter B, Forney J, et al. A randomized controlled pilot study of Outcomes of Strict Allowance of Fluid Therapy in Hyponatremic Heart Failure (SALT-HF). J Card Fail 2013;19(1):1–9.

159. Myung SK, Ju W, Cho B, et al. Efficacy of vitamin and antioxidant supplements in prevention of cardiovascular disease: systematic review and meta-analysis of randomised controlled trials. BMJ 2013;346:f10.

160. Giamouzis G, Kalogeropoulos A, Georgiopoulou V, et al. Hospitalization epidemic in patients with heart failure: risk factors, risk prediction, knowledge gaps, and future directions. J Card Fail 2011; 17(1):54–75.

161. Chaudhry SI, Wang Y, Concato J, et al. Patterns of weight change preceding hospitalization for heart failure. Circulation 2007;116(14):1549–54.

162. Bui AL, Fonarow GC. Home monitoring for heart failure management. J Am Coll Cardiol 2012; 59(2):97–104.

163. Butler J, Subacius H, Vaduganathan M, et al. Relationship between clinical trial site enrollment with participant characteristics, protocol completion, and outcomes: insights From the EVEREST (Efficacy of Vasopressin Antagonism in Heart Failure: outcome Study with Tolvaptan) Trial. J Am Coll Cardiol 2013;61(5):571–9.

164. Blair JE, Khan S, Konstam MA, et al. Weight changes after hospitalization for worsening heart failure and subsequent re-hospitalization and mortality in the EVEREST trial. Eur Heart J 2009;30(13): 1666–73.

165. Piano MR, Prasun MA, Stamos T, et al. Flexible diuretic titration in chronic heart failure: where is the evidence? J Card Fail 2011;17(11):944–54.

166. DeBeradinis B, Januzzi JL Jr. Use of biomarkers to guide outpatient therapy of heart failure. Curr Opin Cardiol 2012;27(6):661–8.

167. Collins SP, Pang PS, Fonarow GC, et al. Is hospital admission for heart failure really necessary?: the role of the emergency department and observation unit in preventing hospitalization and rehospitalization. J Am Coll Cardiol 2013;61(2):121–6.

Optimal Utilization and Management of Implanted Cardiac Rhythm Devices in Patients Hospitalized for Heart Failure

Tiffany Randolph, MD*, Jonathan P. Piccini, MD, MHS

KEYWORDS

- Heart failure • Cardiac resynchronization therapy • Hospitalization

KEY POINTS

- Improved utilization and optimization of device therapy in the management of patients with decompensated heart failure (HF) is an important clinical priority.
- Diagnostic cardiac rhythm device data have been shown to predict hospitalization for HF.
- Cardiac resynchronization therapy (CRT) is a highly effective therapy for the prevention of HF hospitalization.
- Evaluation and optimization of CRT should be considered in all patients admitted with HF despite CRT.
- Optimal device programming is crucial to avoid hospitalization for inappropriate shocks.
- Catheter ablation should be considered in all patients with recurrent implantable cardioverter-defibrillator discharges despite medical therapy.
- The optimal timing of device implantation in patients hospitalized with decompensated heart failure despite medical therapy remains unknown.

Heart failure (HF) affects more than 5.1 million Americans and is responsible for more than one million hospitalizations annually.[1] Multiple studies have shown that in appropriately selected patients with HF, placement of an implantable cardioverter-defibrillator (ICD) decreases the incidence of sudden cardiac death from malignant arrhythmias.[2–4] Furthermore, cardiac resynchronization therapy (CRT) alone or in conjunction with defibrillator therapy (CRT-D) can prevent hospitalizations in patients with HF.[5,6] Most studies to date have focused on the use of these devices in patients with stable symptomatic HF in the outpatient setting. However, given the frequency of HF hospitalizations and growing numbers of patients with ICD or CRT/CRT-D devices, improved utilization and optimization of device therapy in the diagnosis and management of patients with decompensated HF is an important clinical priority.

THE ROLE OF DEVICES IN PREVENTING HOSPITALIZATION

CRT/CRT-D has been shown to reduce hospitalizations and mortality.[7] However, most ICD and CRT devices are also capable of transmitting patient

Division of Cardiology, Duke University Medical Center, 2301 Erwin Road, Durham, NC 27710, USA
* Corresponding author. Electrophysiology Section, Duke University Medical Center, Duke Clinical Research Institute, PO Box 17969, Durham, NC 27710.
E-mail address: tiffany.callaway@duke.edu

Heart Failure Clin 9 (2013) 321–330
http://dx.doi.org/10.1016/j.hfc.2013.04.006
1551-7136/13/$ – see front matter © 2013 Elsevier Inc. All rights reserved.

data to providers remotely, which could be used to prevent HF-related hospitalizations. In patients with chronic HF, symptomatic changes, such as shortness of breath or weight gain, as well physical examination findings, such as rales and edema, often are not detected until the patient is well ensconced in an episode of acutely decompensated heart failure (ADHF). Furthermore, patients with chronic HF may have elevated LV filling pressures without the classic examination or radiographic findings of pulmonary or peripheral edema.[8,9] Therefore, the ability to detect decompensation in clinical status before HF patients become symptomatic is a critical first step in reducing the morbidity, mortality, and health care costs associated with episodes of ADHF.

Changes in intrathoracic impedance have been shown to correlate with episodes of ADHF.[10,11] Simply stated, impedance is the resistance to electrical conductance. As patients develop increasing pulmonary edema, the intrathoracic impedance measured between the right ventricular defibrillation coil and the generator starts to decrease, as current travels more easily through fluid than air.[10–14] Impedance correlates inversely with left ventricular filling pressures and patient weight.[13,14] However, changes in intrathoracic impedance precede the presence of ADHF symptoms by as much as 15 ± 11 days.[13] Device-based impedance data have been used to develop a fluid index algorithm that measures changes in intrathoracic impedance by averaging multiple daily measurements. These values are compared to a reference impedance value obtained 34 days after device implantation.[11] The device records a thoracic impedance fluid index threshold crossing event when there is a consistent negative deviation from the patient's baseline impedance.

Some implantable cardiac devices also use sensed internal electrograms to assess variability in average day and nighttime heart rates. Heart rate variability provides an indirect measure of autonomic tone, as patients with advanced HF often have increased sympathetic nervous system activation coupled with diminished vagal activity. In HF patients, these changes in autonomic activity have been identified as predictors of sudden cardiac death and pump failure.[15,16] Devices can also measure patient activity via a capacitive accelerometer. A decrease in patient activity is a sensitive and objective marker of declining functional capacity. Obviously, all tachytherapy devices record the percentage of ventricular pacing, premature ventricular contraction burden, and episodes of ventricular arrhythmias. Combined with other device-based diagnostics, such as intrathoracic impedance trends, these data provide a wealth of information regarding a patient's status, including information about volume status and electrical stability (arrhythmia burden).

Diagnostic device data have been shown to predict hospitalization. In a cohort of 326 patients with CRT-D devices, decreased intrathoracic impedance and high night heart rate independently predicted hospitalization for HF. In this study, each time a patient's impedance crossed the fluid index threshold, there was a 35% increased risk of HF-associated hospitalizations in the subsequent 4 months (odds ratio 1.352; 95% confidence interval [CI] 1.126 to 1.623, $P<.001$).[11] Subjects without any threshold crossing events were significantly less likely to experience an HF hospitalization in the following 4 months than those with more than 3 threshold crossing events ($P = .001$).

The Program to Access and Review Trending Information and Evaluate Correlation to Symptoms in Patients with Heart Failure (PARTNERS-HF) trial tested the hypothesis that a device-based algorithm could predict episodes of ADHF in patients with CRT-D devices (**Box 1**).[17] Patients judged to be high risk by the algorithm had a 5-fold higher likelihood of being admitted for ADHF during the following 30 days compared with those patients with negative diagnostics (hazard ratio [HR] 5.5; 95% CI 3.4 to 8.8, $P<.0001$). The predictive capacity of the PARTNERS-HF algorithm was not

---

Box 1
PARTNERS-HF device diagnostics algorithm[a]

Fluid index $\geq$100

or 2 of the following:

- Atrial fibrillation $\geq$6 hours in 1 day
- Atrial fibrillation with ventricular rate >90 bpm
- CRT pacing <90% for 5 of 7 days
- High night heart rate
- ICD shock for VT/VF
- Low heart rate variability
- Low patient activity level
- OptiVol Fluid Index $\geq$60

[a] Patients judged to be high risk by the algorithm had a 5-fold higher likelihood of being admitted for ADHF during the following 30 days.

Data from Whellan DJ, Ousdigian KT, Al-Khatib SM, et al. PARTNERS Study Investigators. Combined heart failure device diagnostics identify patients at higher risk of subsequent heart failure hospitalizations: results from PARTNERS HF (Program to Access and Review Trending Information and Evaluate Correlation to Symptoms in Patients With Heart Failure) Study. J Am Coll Cardiol 2010;55:1803–10.

only due to the impedance-based fluid index. A modified algorithm that excluded the fluid index thresholds also indicated increased risk of HF hospitalization.[18]

A pooled analysis from the PARTNERS-HF, OFISSER, FAST, and the CONNECT trials sought to determine if 30-day HF hospitalization readmission could be predicted using device diagnostics.[19] The investigators found that a weighted score based on intrathoracic impedance, atrial fibrillation diagnostics, and nighttime heart rate was able to risk stratify patients as low, moderate, or high risk for repeated HF-related hospitalizations. Patients stratified into the high-risk group were 23 times more likely to be readmitted for HF within 30 days than the low-risk group (HR 22.7; 95% CI 3.2 to 161.7, $P = .002$). At 30 days, 35% were readmitted from the high-risk group compared to 2% in the low-risk group. Risk-stratification systems such as these could be used to better allocate outpatient resources, including postdischarge interventions, toward patients with a higher likelihood of readmission.

Although the above-mentioned technology is readily available in many implanted devices and small trials have shown promise in their ability to predict ADHF and rehospitalization, prospective data are needed to show that interventions based on device diagnostics can decrease hospitalizations or mortality in large populations. Better adoption and utilization of device-based diagnostic algorithms are hindered by limited reimbursement and the considerable resources needed to download and interpret this data in busy hospitals or clinics, which are often already understaffed.

CARDIAC RESYNCHRONIZATION THERAPY

As many as 30% of HF patients have evidence of intraventricular conduction delay and dyssynchronous ventricular contraction.[20] In patients with systolic dysfunction, electrical dyssynchrony further impairs ventricular performance and cardiac output. CRT has been shown to reduce the risk of HF hospitalization and improve quality of life. The MIRACLE trial was the first randomized, double-blind study of CRT. MIRACLE randomized 453 patients with advanced HF (New York Heart Association [NYHA] III-IV), left ventricular ejection fraction (LVEF) less than 35%, and QRS more than 130 ms to CRT versus conventional medical and device therapy. Subjects who received CRT experienced significant improvement in quality-of-life scores (-18.0 vs -9.0 points, $P = .001$), NYHA functional class (-1.0 vs 0.0 class, $P = .001$), 6-min walk distance (+39 vs +10 m, $P = .001$), treadmill exercise time (+81 vs +19 seconds,

$P = .001$), peak V_{O_2} (+1.1 vs +0.1 mL/kg/min, $P = .01$), and LVEF (+4.6 vs -0.2%, $P = .001$). Furthermore, CRT decreased HF hospitalization (7.9% vs 15.1%, HR 0.5; 95% CI 0.28 to 0.84; $P = .02$).[5] In aggregate, trials of CRT in patients with advanced HF have shown a 37% reduction in hospitalization for HF and a 22% reduction in mortality (**Table 1**).[21] Subsequent analysis of the largest CRT trials demonstrated that those with a wider QRS duration (>150 ms) are most likely to benefit from cardiac resynchronization, both in terms of quality of life and in mortality. An analysis of Medicare data demonstrated that compared to patients with a QRS between 120 and 149 ms, patients with a QRS >150 ms had lower 1-year mortality (HR 0.77, 95% CI 0.7 to 0.84, $P<.001$).[22]

Given that the earliest CRT studies focused on patients with NYHA III and IV HF, MADIT-CRT sought to discern whether the same benefits in hospitalization and quality of life would be obtained in patients with less severe symptoms. In patients with mild HF (NYHA class I or II), LVEF <30%, and a QRS duration $\geq$130 ms, CRT-D led to a significant reduction in the composite primary endpoint of all-cause mortality or HF-related events (HR 0.66; 95% CI 0.52 to 0.84; $P = 0001$). Although there were no statistically significant differences in all-cause mortality between groups, there was a striking reduction (41%) in HF events.[23]

Based on the available evidence, the 2012 American College of Cardiology Foundation/American Heart Association/Heart Rhythm Society Focused Update of the 2008 Guidelines for Device-Based Therapy[24] provide a class I recommendation for CRT inpatients with left bundle branch block, QRS $\geq$ 150 ms, LVEF $\leq$ 35%, and NYHA class II-IV symptoms despite optimal medical therapy. The guidelines also provide a level IIa recommendation for the same patients if the QRS is 120 to 149 (Level of Evidence B) or if there is a non-left bundle branch block, QRS $\geq$ 150 ms, and NYHA III-IV symptoms (Level of Evidence A). Finally, the guidelines also stress the importance of a collaborative approach between HF, electrophysiology, and imaging specialists to ensure that medications, device parameters, and device placement are optimized.[25]

MANAGEMENT OF IMPLANTABLE DEVICES DURING AN ADMISSION FOR HF

The American College of Cardiology/American Heart Association/Heart Rhythm Society guidelines for follow-up of ICD and CRT-D devices recommend in-person follow-up within 72 hours of implantation and again 2 to 12 weeks after implantation. Following these initial follow-up visits,

Table 1
Reduction in hospitalization in major trials of cardiac resynchronization

Trial	Year	N	Population	Intervention	Endpoint	Treatment Effect
MUSTIC[5]	2001	67	NYHA III, QRS ≥150 ms	CRT vs VVI 40	HF hospitalizations	4.5% vs 13.4%; P<.05
CONTAK[49]	2003	490	NYHA II to IV HF, EF ≤35%, QRS >120 ms	CRT-D vs CRT off +ICD	HF hospitalizations	13.1% vs 15.9%
MIRACLE-ICD[50]	2003	369	NYHA III/IV, EF ≤35%, QRS >130 ms	CRT-D vs CRT off +ICD	HF hospitalizations	45.5% vs 42.9%
COMPANION[51]	2004	1520	NYHA III/IV, QRS ≥120 ms	Medical therapy vs CRT-P vs CRT-D	All-cause mortality or hospitalizations	CRT HR 0.75; 95% CI 0.63 to 0.90, P = .002 CRT-D HR 0.72; 95% CI 0.60 to 0.86, P<.001
MIRACLE-ICD II[52]	2004	186	NYHA II HF, EF ≤35%, QRS ≥130 ms	CRT-D vs CRT off +ICD	Mortality or HF hospitalization	25.9% vs 25.7%; P = .69
CARE-HF[53]	2005	813	NYHA III/IV, EF ≤35%, QRS ≥120 ms, LVEDD ≥30 mm	CRT vs medical therapy	HF hospitalizations	17.6% vs 32.9%; HR 0.48; 95% CI 0.36 to 0.64, P<.001
REVERSE[54]	2008	610	NYHA I/II, EF ≤40%, QRS ≥120 ms	CRT on vs CRT off	HF hospitalizations	7.3% vs 2.9%; HR 0.47, P = .03
MADIT-CRT[23]	2009	1820	NYHA I/II, EF ≤30%, QRS ≥130 ms	CRT-D vs ICD	HF events	13.9% vs 22.8%; HR 0.59; 95% CI 0.47 to 0.74, P<.001
RAFT[55]	2010	1798	NYHA II/III, EF ≤30%, QRS ≥120 ms or paced QRS >200 ms	CRT-D vs ICD	HF hospitalizations	19.5% vs 26.1%; HR 0.68; 95% CI 0.56 to 0.83, P<.001

the guidelines recommend annual in-clinic follow-up, supplemented with in-clinic or remote interrogation every 6 months.[26] Although the guidelines acknowledge that more frequent follow-up may be necessary if clinically indicated, there are no specific recommendations regarding what clinical events constitute the need for more frequent monitoring. Implanted cardiac rhythm devices should be interrogated in the event of an ICD firing or when patients develop symptoms that may be attributable to an arrhythmia. However, devices may also provide useful information following HF hospitalization. On interrogation, the provider may be able to determine if ventricular arrhythmia/ectopy, or poorly rate-controlled atrial fibrillation/flutter, may have contributed to the current episode of ADHF.

Arguably, patients with a CRT/CRT-D device who are hospitalized with decompensated HF may represent CRT nonresponders and, therefore, should at least have their devices interrogated during their hospitalization, if not optimized. In patients with CRT or CRT-D, an evaluation of their biventricular pacing may also help identify the cause for their decompensation. If the percentage of biventricular pacing is less than 90% to 95%, the reasons for low pacing burden should be identified and corrected (**Fig. 1**). This may include improved rate control in patients with atrial fibrillation, suppression of premature ventricular ectopy, or optimization of the atrioventricular and interventricular timing. Finally, the position of the coronary sinus lead should also be assessed with chest radiograph. The MADIT-CRT study found that LV apical pacing was associated with a higher risk of death or progressive HF (HR 1.72, 95% CI 1.09 to 2.71, $P = .019$). If the coronary sinus lead position is anterior or apical, strong consideration should be given to revising the lead location, particularly if the patient has never experienced an improvement in LV function or symptoms after implantation.

Suboptimal atrioventricular timing and contraction lead to reduced ventricular filling time, decreased preload, and, ultimately, reduced cardiac output. The goal of atrioventricular (AV) optimization is to identify the AV delay that allows for maximal LV filling before the onset of systole. Prolonged VV relationships occur when there is a delay between right ventricular and LV activation and subsequent interventricular dyssynchrony. Several clinical trials have evaluated the efficacy of AV and VV optimization in outpatients with HF. The Frequent Optimization Study Using the QuickOpt Method (FREEDOM) and SmartDelay determined AV Optimization (SMART AV) trials demonstrated that routine optimization of AV and VV timing did not lead to significant improvement in clinical outcomes or functional status.[27,28] However, it remains unclear whether optimization can improve outcomes in CRT nonresponders and those hospitalized with HF.

An open question is whether patients with CRT devices who are admitted with ADHF should undergo optimization as a matter of routine. Mullens and colleagues[29] analyzed a group of 75 CRT nonresponders and discovered that after addressing reversible factors, such as uncontrolled arrhythmias, anemia, suboptimal medical therapy, and poor LV lead position, AV optimization led to statistically significant improvements in LVEF, LV filling, quality of life, and 6-min walk. Given the burden of rehospitalization for HF, a trial evaluating CRT optimization, including AV and VV optimization in those with ADHF, would address an interesting and clinically relevant hypothesis.

INPATIENT MANAGEMENT OF PATIENTS WHO PRESENT WITH A SHOCK

Between 25% and 32% of HF patients with primary prevention ICDs will experience an ICD discharge within 1 to 3 years of implantation.[30,31] The timing and appropriate location for evaluation of these patients depends on the clinical scenario, including whether the therapy was appropriate or inappropriate.[31,32] In either scenario, patients need prompt evaluation to determine the inciting cause and to institute appropriate preventive interventions. Patients who experience one isolated firing of their ICD and are free of symptoms such as progressive HF or ischemia can safely be evaluated in the outpatient setting within 1 week of the event.[33,34] Many centers, including the authors' center, prefer to evaluate these patients within 48 hours of the event. However, those with symptoms or those who experience more than one shock should be evaluated in clinic within 24 hours or seen in the emergency department immediately. Remote monitoring greatly facilitates rapid triage and evaluation.

After ascertaining the patient's recent history to identify potential reasons for ICD firing (eg, ischemic chest pain), the device should be interrogated. This interrogation can help differentiate appropriate and inappropriate shocks as well as determine if the patient is in electrical storm (3 or more shocks in 24 hours). Up to 10% to 20% of all ICD shocks in primary and secondary prevention patients are inappropriate,[2,31,32,35] often due to atrial fibrillation, atrial flutter, or supraventricular tachycardia.[30–32] Other potential causes of inappropriate ICD therapy include oversensing of T waves or diaphragmatic myopotentials, electromagnetic

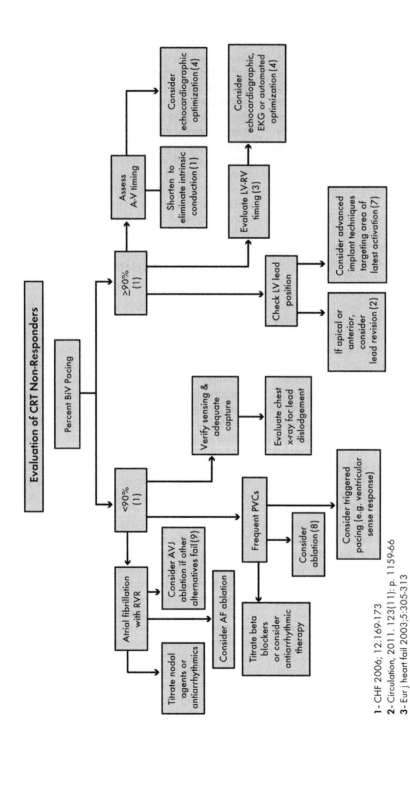

Fig. 1. Evaluation of CRT nonresponders.

1 - CHF 2006; 12:169-173
2 - Circulation, 2011. 123(11): p. 1159-66
3 - Eur j heart fail 2003;5:305-313
4 - J Cardiovasc Electrophysiol 2012;23:110-118
5 - CHF 2006;12:219-222
6 - Am J Cardiol 2002;89:198-203
7 - J Am Coll Cardiol. 2010;56:774-781
8 - J Cardiovasc Electrophysiol 2008;19:708-715
9 - Heart Rhythm 2010;7:1240-1245

interference, or mechanical failure, such as lead fracture, or insulation breaks. The most important step in preventing inappropriate shocks is the use of optimal ICD programming. In patients with primary prevention ICDs, liberalized detection algorithms with delayed detection and higher detection thresholds have been shown to lead to improved survival.[36,37]

In patients who present with appropriate shocks for ventricular arrhythmias, the first step is to assess and treat any potential reversible causes, such as electrolyte disturbances, ischemia, or HF exacerbations. For HF patients with refractory episodes of sustained ventricular tachyarrhythmias, pharmacologic options are somewhat limited. Because β-blockade has been proven to reduce mortality in the HF population, a reasonable first step is titrating β-blockade as tolerated. Although acute β-blocker therapy is usually administered with intravenous metoprolol or esmolol, accumulating evidence suggests that carvedilol may have superior antiarrhythmic properties compared to other β-blockers.[38–40]

The only pharmacologic agent recommended in the American College of Cardiology/American Heart Association guidelines for the treatment of ventricular arrhythmias in patients with HF is amiodarone.[41] The SCD-HeFT trial did not show a significant increase in mortality with this drug compared to placebo.[2] However, acute antiarrhythmic therapy with lidocaine is a reasonable first step, particularly if a patient has ischemic cardiomyopathy. Procainamide is another effective medication for acute arrhythmia control. If antiarrhythmic therapy is not immediately successful in patients with ventricular storm, intubation and sedation should be performed until the arrhythmic storm is controlled. Catheter ablation is an increasingly used treatment for recurrent or refractory ventricular arrhythmias. Several clinical trials have demonstrated that catheter ablation results in superior shock reduction compared with medical therapy alone.[42,43] Investigational therapies, such as sympathectomy, vagal stimulation, and perhaps even renal denervation, may also play a role pending evaluation in clinical trials.

OPTIMAL TIMING OF DEVICE IMPLANTATION

Another important question in patients who are hospitalized for HF is the optimal timing of implantation of ICD or CRT-D devices. In patients with ischemic cardiomyopathy, several clinical trials have addressed ICD implantation early after myocardial infarction. The Defibrillator in Acute Myocardial Infarction Trial (DINAMIT) demonstrated that in patients with a recent myocardial infarction and an ejection fraction of less than 35%, there was no survival advantage in placement of an ICD sooner than 40 days after their myocardial infarction (HR 1.08, 95% CI 0.96 to 1.08, $P = .66$). Although there was a decreased incidence of death secondary to arrhythmia in the ICD arm (3.6% vs 8.5% in the control group, HR 0.42; 95% CI 0.22–0.83), there was also an increase in nonarrhythmic death in those who received an ICD (15.1% vs 8.5%, HR 1.75; 95% CI 1.11–2.76). The more recent IRIS study supports the findings of DINAMIT.[44] Whether noninvasive interventions such as the wearable external defibrillator have a role remains to be seen.[45]

In patients with chronic HF on optimal medical therapy who are admitted for an exacerbation or progression of their HF, the data on optimal timing of device placement are less clear.[41] There are no guidelines as to when device implantation should occur in eligible patients with a recent hospitalization. Ajijola and colleagues[46] attempted to address this question by retrospectively analyzing patients who received a CRT device as an inpatient compared to those whose devices were implanted as outpatients. The inpatients were admitted for ADHF, arrhythmia, syncope, or non-ST elevation myocardial infarction. The investigators discovered that those whose devices were implanted as inpatients were more likely to be readmitted with episodes of ADHF within 2 years following implant (HR 1.6; 95% CI 1.03 to 2.48, $P = .038$). However, after using propensity scores to adjust for the baseline differences between groups, there were no statistically significant differences in HF hospitalizations or the combined end point of HF hospitalizations, all-cause mortality, left ventricular assist device placement, or cardiac transplant. These findings suggest that the increased incidence of hospitalization associated with inpatient implantation was likely attributable to differences in comorbidities, such as diabetes, renal insufficiency, and HF severity, rather than the timing of CRT-D implantation.

Although prospective studies have failed to reveal a survival or hospitalization benefit to early implantation, the Organized Program to Initiate Lifesaving Treatment in Hospitalized Patients with Heart Failure retrospectively analyzed 4685 patients with LVEF $\leq$35% who were eligible for an ICD and found that only 8% received an ICD during their hospitalization. That group's mortality was 38.1% compared to 52.3% in those who did not receive an ICD as an inpatient ($P<.001$).[47] Recognizing that these are retrospective studies and are limited by bias and confounding, larger prospective studies are needed to define the optimal window of implantation in patients who are in decompensated HF. The limited data that are currently available do not yet provide any convincing evidence to guide clinicians with this decision. In patients who have not yet received an opportunity for improvement in LVEF by optimization of medical therapy, it is reasonable to wait 1 to 3 months before device implementation. However, in those who are deemed at extreme risk of SCD in the time interval between discharge and reevaluation for device placement, a wearable cardioverter-defibrillator vest may be a viable option.[48]

SUMMARY

Implantable cardiac rhythm devices have an important and proven role in the treatment of chronic stable HF and prevention of HF hospitalizations. Less is known about the utility of devices for predicting and avoiding episodes of decompensated HF. Large, prospective trials are needed to elucidate fully the potential role and cost of adopting remote monitoring to prevent HF hospitalization. In addition, prospective studies are also needed to help clarify the optimal timing of device therapy in patients with decompensated HF. Although ICD and CRT therapy are landmark advances in the treatment of HF, more work is needed to realize their full potential.

REFERENCES

1. Epstein AE, DiMarco JP, Ellenbogen KA, et al. 2012 ACCF/AHA/HRS focused update incorporated into the ACCF/AHA/HRS 2008 guidelines for device-based therapy of cardiac rhythm abnormalities: a report of the American College of Cardiology Foundation/American Heart Association Task Force on Practice Guidelines and the Heart Rhythm Society. Circulation 2013;127:e283–352.
2. Bardy GH, Lee KL, Mark DB, et al. Amiodarone or an implantable cardioverter-defibrillator for congestive heart failure. N Engl J Med 2005; 352(3):225–37.
3. Moss AJ, Hall WJ, Cannom DS, et al. Improved survival with an implanted defibrillator in patients with coronary disease at high risk for ventricular arrhythmia. Multicenter Automatic Defibrillator Implantation Trial Investigators. N Engl J Med 1996; 335(26):1933–40.
4. Moss AJ, Zareba W, Hall WJ, et al. Prophylactic implantation of a defibrillator in patients with myocardial infarction and reduced ejection fraction. N Engl J Med 2002;346(12):877–83.
5. Abraham WT, Fisher WG, Smith AL, et al. Cardiac resynchronization in chronic heart failure. N Engl J Med 2002;346(24):1845–53.
6. Bristow MR, Feldman AM, Saxon LA. Heart failure management using implantable devices for ventricular resynchronization: comparison of Medical Therapy, Pacing, and Defibrillation in Chronic Heart Failure (COMPANION) trial. COMPANION Steering Committee and COMPANION Clinical Investigators. J Card Fail 2000;6(3):276–85.
7. Al-Majed NS, McAlister FA, Bakal JA, et al. Meta-analysis: cardiac resynchronization therapy for patients with less symptomatic heart failure. Ann Intern Med 2011;154(6):401–12.
8. Stevenson LW, Perloff JK. The limited reliability of physical signs for estimating hemodynamics in chronic heart failure. JAMA 1989;261(6):884–8.
9. Mahdyoon H, Klein R, Eyler W, et al. Radiographic pulmonary congestion in end-stage congestive heart failure. Am J Cardiol 1989;63(9):625–7.
10. Catanzariti D, Lunati M, Landolina M, et al. Monitoring intrathoracic impedance with an implantable defibrillator reduces hospitalizations in patients with heart failure. Pacing Clin Electrophysiol 2009; 32(3):363–70.
11. Small RS, Wickemeyer W, Germany R, et al. Changes in intrathoracic impedance are associated with subsequent risk of hospitalizations for acute decompensated heart failure: clinical utility of implanted device monitoring without a patient alert. J Card Fail 2009;15(6):475–81.
12. Ypenburg C, Bax JJ, van der Wall EE, et al. Intrathoracic impedance monitoring to predict decompensated heart failure. Am J Cardiol 2007;99(4): 554–7.
13. Yu CM, Wang L, Chau E, et al. Intrathoracic impedance monitoring in patients with heart failure: correlation with fluid status and feasibility of early warning preceding hospitalization. Circulation 2005;112(6):841–8.
14. Abraham WT, Compton S, Haas G, et al. Intrathoracic impedance vs daily weight monitoring for predicting worsening heart failure events: results of the Fluid Accumulation Status Trial (FAST). Congest Heart Fail 2011;17(2):51–5.
15. Bilchick KC, Fetics B, Djoukeng R, et al. Prognostic value of heart rate variability in chronic congestive heart failure (Veterans Affairs' Survival Trial of Antiarrhythmic Therapy in Congestive Heart Failure). Am J Cardiol 2002;90(1):24–8.
16. Bilchick KC, Berger RD. Heart rate variability. J Cardiovasc Electrophysiol 2006;17(6):691–4.
17. Whellan DJ, Ousdigian KT, Al-Khatib SM, et al. Combined heart failure device diagnostics identify patients at higher risk of subsequent heart failure hospitalizations: results from PARTNERS HF (Program to Access and Review Trending Information and Evaluate Correlation to Symptoms in Patients With Heart Failure) study. J Am Coll Cardiol 2010; 55(17):1803–10.

18. Sarkar S, Koehler J, Crossley GH, et al. Burden of atrial fibrillation and poor rate control detected by continuous monitoring and the risk for heart failure hospitalization. Am Heart J 2012;164(4):616–24.

19. Whellan DJ, Sarkar S, Koehler J, et al. Development of a method to risk stratify patients with heart failure for 30-day readmission using implantable device diagnostics. Am J Cardiol 2013;111(1): 79–84.

20. Leclercq C, Kass DA. Retiming the failing heart: principles and current clinical status of cardiac resynchronization. J Am Coll Cardiol 2002;39(2): 194–201.

21. McAlister FA, Ezekowitz J, Hooton N, et al. Cardiac resynchronization therapy for patients with left ventricular systolic dysfunction: a systematic review. JAMA 2007;297(22):2502–14.

22. Bilchick KC, Kamath S, DiMarco JP, et al. Bundle-branch block morphology and other predictors of outcome after cardiac resynchronization therapy in Medicare patients. Circulation 2010;122(20): 2022–30.

23. Moss AJ, Hall WJ, Cannom DS, et al. Cardiac-resynchronization therapy for the prevention of heart-failure events. N Engl J Med 2009;361(14): 1329–38.

24. Epstein AE, DiMarco JP, Ellenbogen KA, et al. 2012 ACCF/AHA/HRS focused update incorporated into the ACCF/AHA/HRS 2008 guidelines for device-based therapy of cardiac rhythm abnormalities: a report of the American College of Cardiology Foundation/American Heart Association Task Force on Practice Guidelines and the Heart Rhythm Society. J Am Coll Cardiol 2013;61(3):e6–75.

25. Francis GS, Greenberg BH, Hsu DT, et al. ACCF/AHA/ACP/HFSA/ISHLT 2010 clinical competence statement on management of patients with advanced heart failure and cardiac transplant: a report of the ACCF/AHA/ACP Task Force on Clinical Competence and Training. Circulation 2010;122(6): 644–72.

26. Tracy CM, Epstein AE, Darbar D, et al. 2012 ACCF/AHA/HRS focused update of the 2008 guidelines for device-based therapy of cardiac rhythm abnormalities: a report of the American College of Cardiology Foundation/American Heart Association Task Force on Practice Guidelines and the Heart Rhythm Society. Circulation 2012;126(14):1784–800.

27. Abraham WT, Gras D, Yu CM, et al. Rationale and design of a randomized clinical trial to assess the safety and efficacy of frequent optimization of cardiac resynchronization therapy: the Frequent Optimization Study Using the QuickOpt Method (FREEDOM) trial. Am Heart J 2010;159(6): 944–948.e1.

28. Ellenbogen KA, Gold MR, Meyer TE, et al. Primary results from the SmartDelay determined AV optimization: a comparison to other AV delay methods used in cardiac resynchronization therapy (SMART-AV) trial: a randomized trial comparing empirical, echocardiography-guided, and algorithmic atrioventricular delay programming in cardiac resynchronization therapy. Circulation 2010; 122(25):2660–8.

29. Mullens W, Grimm RA, Verga T, et al. Insights from a cardiac resynchronization optimization clinic as part of a heart failure disease management program. J Am Coll Cardiol 2009;53(9):765–73.

30. Poole JE, Johnson GW, Hellkamp AS, et al. Prognostic importance of defibrillator shocks in patients with heart failure. N Engl J Med 2008;359(10): 1009–17.

31. Daubert JP, Zareba W, Cannom DS, et al. Inappropriate implantable cardioverter-defibrillator shocks in MADIT II: frequency, mechanisms, predictors, and survival impact. J Am Coll Cardiol 2008; 51(14):1357–65.

32. Klein RC, Raitt MH, Wilkoff BL, et al. Analysis of implantable cardioverter defibrillator therapy in the Antiarrhythmics Versus Implantable Defibrillators (AVID) Trial. J Cardiovasc Electrophysiol 2003; 14(9):940–8.

33. Gehi AK, Mehta D, Gomes JA. Evaluation and management of patients after implantable cardioverter-defibrillator shock. JAMA 2006;296(23):2839–47.

34. Sears SF Jr, Shea JB, Conti JB. Cardiology patient page. How to respond to an implantable cardioverter-defibrillator shock. Circulation 2005; 111(23):e380–2.

35. Kadish A, Dyer A, Daubert JP, et al. Prophylactic defibrillator implantation in patients with nonischemic dilated cardiomyopathy. N Engl J Med 2004; 350(21):2151–8.

36. Moss AJ, Schuger C, Beck CA, et al. Reduction in inappropriate therapy and mortality through ICD programming. N Engl J Med 2012;367(24): 2275–83.

37. Wilkoff BL, Williamson BD, Stern RS, et al. Strategic programming of detection and therapy parameters in implantable cardioverter-defibrillators reduces shocks in primary prevention patients: results from the PREPARE (Primary Prevention Parameters Evaluation) study. J Am Coll Cardiol 2008;52(7):541–50.

38. Gattis WA, O'Connor CM, Leimberger JD, et al. Clinical outcomes in patients on beta-blocker therapy admitted with worsening chronic heart failure. Am J Cardiol 2003;91(2):169–74.

39. Fonarow GC. Role of in-hospital initiation of carvedilol to improve treatment rates and clinical outcomes. Am J Cardiol 2004;93(9A):77B–81B.

40. Thattassery E, Gheorghiade M. Beta blocker therapy after acute myocardial infarction in patients with heart failure and systolic dysfunction. Heart Fail Rev 2004;9(2):107–13.

41. Jessup M, Abraham WT, Casey DE, et al. 2009 focused update: ACCF/AHA Guidelines for the Diagnosis and Management of Heart Failure in Adults: a report of the American College of Cardiology Foundation/American Heart Association Task Force on Practice Guidelines: developed in collaboration with the International Society for Heart and Lung Transplantation. Circulation 2009;119(14):1977–2016.

42. Reddy VY, Reynolds MR, Neuzil P, et al. Prophylactic catheter ablation for the prevention of defibrillator therapy. N Engl J Med 2007;357(26):2657–65.

43. Kuck KH, Schaumann A, Eckardt L, et al. Catheter ablation of stable ventricular tachycardia before defibrillator implantation in patients with coronary heart disease (VTACH): a multicentre randomised controlled trial. Lancet 2010;375(9708):31–40.

44. Steinbeck G, Andresen D, Seidl K, et al. Defibrillator implantation early after myocardial infarction. N Engl J Med 2009;361(15):1427–36.

45. Health, U.S.N.I.o. Vest Prevention of Early Sudden Death Trial and VEST Registry. 2013 [cited 2013 March 28]. Available at: http://clinicaltrials.gov/ct2/show/NCT01446965?term=VEST&rank=1. Accesed April 16, 2013.

46. Ajijola OA, Macklin EA, Moore SA, et al. Inpatient vs. elective outpatient cardiac resynchronization therapy device implantation and long-term clinical outcome. Europace 2010;12(12):1745–9.

47. Hernandez AF, Fonarow GC, Hammill BG, et al. Clinical effectiveness of implantable cardioverter-defibrillators among medicare beneficiaries with heart failure. Circ Heart Fail 2010;3(1):7–13.

48. Chung MK, Szymkiewicz SJ, Shao M, et al. Aggregate national experience with the wearable cardioverter-defibrillator: event rates, compliance,

and survival. J Am Coll Cardiol 2010;56(3): 194–203.

49. Higgins SL, Hummel JD, Niazi IK, et al. Cardiac resynchronization therapy for the treatment of heart failure in patients with intraventricular conduction delay and malignant ventricular tachyarrhythmias. J Am Coll Cardiol 2003;42(8):1454–9.

50. Young JB, Abraham WT, Smith AL, et al. Combined cardiac resynchronization and implantable cardioversion defibrillation in advanced chronic heart failure: the MIRACLE ICD Trial. JAMA 2003;289(20): 2685–94.

51. Bristow MR, Saxon LA, Boehmer J, et al. Cardiac-resynchronization therapy with or without an implantable defibrillator in advanced chronic heart failure. N Engl J Med 2004;350(21):2140–50.

52. Abraham WT, Young JB, Leon AR, et al. Effects of cardiac resynchronization on disease progression in patients with left ventricular systolic dysfunction, an indication for an implantable cardioverter-defibrillator, and mildly symptomatic chronic heart failure. Circulation 2004;110(18):2864–8.

53. Cleland JG, Daubert JC, Erdmann E, et al. The effect of cardiac resynchronization on morbidity and mortality in heart failure. N Engl J Med 2005; 352(15):1539–49.

54. Linde C, Abraham WT, Gold MR, et al. Randomized trial of cardiac resynchronization in mildly symptomatic heart failure patients and in asymptomatic patients with left ventricular dysfunction and previous heart failure symptoms. J Am Coll Cardiol 2008;52(23):1834–43.

55. Tang AS, Wells GA, Talajic M, et al. Cardiac-resynchronization therapy for mild-to-moderate heart failure. N Engl J Med 2010;363(25): 2385–95.

The Potential Role of Nonpharmacologic Electrophysiology-Based Interventions in Improving Outcomes in Patients Hospitalized for Heart Failure

Norman C. Wang, MD[a], Jonathan P. Piccini, MD, MHS[b],
Gregg C. Fonarow, MD[c], Bradley P. Knight, MD[d],
Matthew E. Harinstein, MD[a], Javed Butler, MD, MPH[e],
Marc K. Lahiri, MD[f], Marco Metra, MD[g],
Muthiah Vaduganathan, MD, MPH[h], Mihai Gheorghiade, MD[i],*

KEYWORDS

- Electrophysiology • Heart failure • Hospitalization • Outcomes

KEY POINTS

- Hospitalization for heart failure (HHF) syndromes have high postdischarge mortality and morbidity.
- Few interventions during or soon after hospitalization improve long-term outcomes in HHF.
- Nonpharmacologic electrophysiology-based interventions have a significant impact on outpatients with chronic heart failure, but the role of these therapies in patients with HHF is largely unknown because of lack of systematic investigation.
- The optimal timing of these interventions in the postdischarge period is not well defined.
- Future studies are needed to clarify mechanisms behind worsening heart failure and the potential role of electrophysiologic therapies, given the poor outcomes.

INTRODUCTION

Heart failure is an epidemic in industrialized nations.[1] In the United States, there were more than 1 million admissions in 2009.[2] It is the most frequent cause of hospital admissions and readmissions among older adults.[3,4] Compounding the scope of this problem, a hospitalization for heart

Disclosures: See last page of article.

[a] Heart and Vascular Institute, University of Pittsburgh Medical Center, 200 Lothrop Street, Pittsburgh, PA 15213, USA; [b] Division of Cardiology, Duke Clinical Research Institute, Duke University Medical Center, PO Box 17969, Durham, NC 27705, USA; [c] Ahmanson-UCLA Cardiomyopathy Center, Ronald Reagan UCLA Medical Center, 10833 LeConte Avenue, Room A2-237 CHS, Los Angeles, CA 90095, USA; [d] Northwestern University Feinberg School of Medicine, 251 East Huron Street, Feinberg 8-503E, Chicago, IL 60611, USA; [e] Division of Cardiology, Department of Medicine, Emory Cardiovascular Clinical Research Institute, 1462 Clifton Road NE, Suite 504, Atlanta, GA 30322, USA; [f] Edith and Benson Ford Heart and Vascular Institute, Department of Internal Medicine, Henry Ford Hospital, 2799 West Grand Boulevard, Detroit, MI 48202, USA; [g] Cardiology, Department of Medical and Surgical Specialties, Radiological Sciences and Public Health, University of Brescia, Piazza Spedali Civili 1, 25123, Brescia, Italy; [h] Department of Medicine, Massachusetts General Hospital, 55 Fruit Street, GRB 740, Boston, MA 02114, USA; [i] Center for Cardiovascular Innovation, Northwestern University Feinberg School of Medicine, 645 North Michigan Avenue, Suite 1006, Chicago, IL 60611, USA
* Corresponding author.
E-mail address: m-gheorghiade@northwestern.edu

Heart Failure Clin 9 (2013) 331–343
http://dx.doi.org/10.1016/j.hfc.2013.04.007
1551-7136/13/$ – see front matter © 2013 Elsevier Inc. All rights reserved.

failure (HHF) is associated with a 60-day to 90-day postdischarge mortality and rehospitalization rate of up to 15% and 30%, respectively.[5] It is one of the most important predictors of outcome in those with chronic heart failure.[6]

Patients with HHF encompass a heterogeneous spectrum, which can be divided into 3 main groups.[5] The first are those with new-onset or first-detected heart failure. The second group consists of patients with chronic heart failure admitted with exacerbation. These acutely decompensated patients represent most patients with HHF. The third group has end-stage heart failure. Unless offered a transplant or a ventricular assist device, many of these patients with end-stage heart failure often benefit from palliative care consultation.

For those who survive to be discharged, optimization of evidenced-based medications is recommended, because many eligible patients do not receive them.[7] Registry data indicate that angiotensin-converting enzyme inhibitors, angiotensin-receptor blockers, β-blockers, and aldosterone antagonists are associated with lower readmission rates in patients with reduced left ventricular ejection fraction (LVEF).[8,9] Some patients have good prognosis with medical treatment alone and transition to stable, chronic heart failure. Despite optimal medical therapy, approximately half are readmitted within the next 6 months.[10] These poor outcomes have persisted despite therapeutic advances (**Fig. 1**).[11] Recurrent heart rhythm disorders may be primary exacerbating

factors for rehospitalization and prevent complete recovery from initial decompensation. Certain patients may benefit from early nonpharmacologic interventions to cross a threshold for recovery.

Patients with chronic heart failure generally exist in the stable outpatient setting and in the HHF setting. For outpatients with reduced LVEF, numerous randomized trials have shown improved outcomes with pharmacologic and nonpharmacologic therapies and are the basis for clinical guidelines.[12–14] These evidence-based therapies are effective in real-world clinical practice.[15] In contrast, no specific therapy has been shown to improve outcomes after HHF in randomized clinical trials. Targeting heart rhythm disorders with nonpharmacologic electrophysiology-based interventions represents a significant opportunity. Recent American College of Cardiology/American Heart Association and European Society of Cardiology guidelines contain new sections for the hospitalized patient and appropriately identified atrial and ventricular arrhythmias as potential targets for therapy.[12,16] Further recommendations on how to apply nonpharmacologic electrophysiology-based interventions in the setting are not presented, highlighting the paucity of data (**Table 1**).

The pathophysiology leading to HHF syndromes is often multifactorial and remains an intense area of investigation. Nonetheless, those who are discharged have similar modes of death as those with stable outpatient heart failure, albeit at higher rates.[17] Thus, patients with HHF may derive a larger

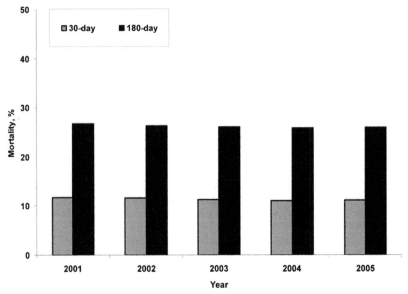

Fig. 1. Mortality at 30 and 180 days after discharge from heart failure hospitalization in Medicare beneficiaries between 2001 and 2005. (*Data from* Curtis LH, Greiner MA, Hammill BG, et al. Early and long-term outcomes of heart failure in elderly persons, 2001–2005. Arch Intern Med 2008;168:2483.)

Table 1
Nonpharmacologic electrophysiology-based interventions addressed in 2009 American College of Cardiology Foundation/America Heart Association Heart Failure Guidelines

Heart Rhythm Disorder	Intervention	Chronic Heart Failure		HHF	
		Preserved LVEF	Reduced LVEF	Preserved LVEF	Reduced LVEF
Sinus node dysfunction	Non-CRT pacemaker	T	T	N	N
Atrioventricular block	Non-CRT pacemaker	T	T	N	N
	CRT	R	R	N	N
Cardiac dyssynchrony	CRT	N	R	N	N
Atrial fibrillation	Pacemaker + AVN ablation	T	T	N	N
	Pulmonary vein isolation	T	T	N	N
Atrial flutter	Catheter Ablation	N	N	N	N
Paroxysmal SVT	Catheter Ablation	N	N	N	N
Ventricular Tachycardia	ICD	N	R	N	N
	Catheter Ablation	N	N	N	N
Ventricular Fibrillation	ICD	N	R	N	N
	Catheter Ablation	N	N	N	N

Abbreviations: AVN, atrioventricular node; CRT, cardiac resynchronization therapy; ICD, implantable cardioverter-defibrillator; N, not addressed in guidelines; R, recommendation given in guidelines; SVT, supraventricular tachycardia; T, addressed in guidelines text without recommendation.

absolute benefit from interventions with lower numbers needed to treat. However, net benefit in 1 clinical setting does not necessarily translate into benefit at a different phase in the natural history of a given disorder. Patients who stabilize after discharge should be considered patients with chronic stable heart failure and treated as such, but it is unclear what objective measurements may quantify that transition.[18]

Heart failure and heart rhythm disorders have a complex interaction (**Fig. 2**). Many patients with HHF would clearly be appropriate candidates for nonpharmacologic electrophysiology-based interventions if their indications were identified in the stable outpatient setting. All too often they come to attention by virtue of being hospitalized. Although procedural-related risks are higher in the setting of acute illness, earlier intervention may also lead to substantial downstream benefit, which would otherwise have not be realized. The purpose of this article is to explore the use of nonpharmacologic electrophysiology-based interventions and how they may be applied in the HHF setting in addition to optimal medical therapy. Areas of need for future research and innovation (**Box 1**) to improve outcomes in this epidemic are also highlighted.

Implantable Cardioverter-Defibrillators

Implantable cardioverter-defibrillator (ICD) therapy for primary prevention of sudden death in heart failure is confined to outpatients with chronically reduced LVEF who have been on optimal medical therapy for heart failure for several months.[19] Randomized trials support the mortality benefit for those with ischemic and nonischemic cause and mild to moderate symptoms.[20,21] Despite the effectiveness of ICDs in treating ventricular arrhythmias, there is concern for deleterious effects, including an increased risk of heart failure events after ICD shocks.[22,23] Moreover, ICD shocks do not necessarily correlate with aborted sudden death.[24,25] It has been hypothesized that ICD shocks cause myocardial injury and contribute to the progression of underlying cardiac dysfunction. A high percentage of right ventricular pacing may also contribute to worsening heart failure.[26] Because of these and other concerns, some recommend postdischarge outpatient reevaluation to assess ICD candidacy.[27]

Data supporting insertion of an ICD at the time of HHF or in the early postdischarge period are limited. A study of Medicare beneficiaries aged 65 years and older with HFF[28] showed that ICD

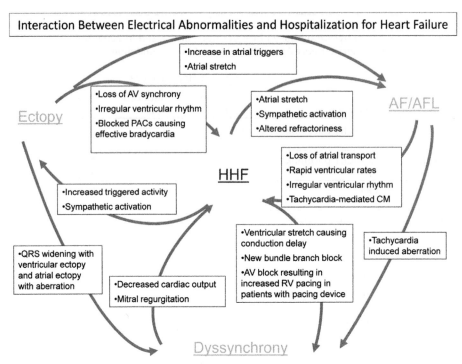

Fig. 2. Potential interactions between heart rhythm disorders and HHF syndromes. AF, atrial fibrillation; AFL, atrial flutter; AV, atrioventricular; CM, cardiomyopathy; PACs, premature atrial complexes; RV, right ventricular.

placement is associated with lower mortality at 3 years (38.1% vs 52.3%, P<.001) (**Fig. 3**). Given the retrospective design and possibility of residual confounding, these findings need to be replicated in a prospective randomized clinical trial. In contrast, data from an acute heart failure trial[29] showed that the presence of an ICD at HHF admission is associated with no overall mortality benefit and increased postdischarge hospitalizations, despite a trend toward reduction in sudden death (hazard ratio, 0.66, 95% confidence interval, 0.43–1.02). Possible reasons for lack of ICD benefit include competing risk from heart failure death, and mechanisms of sudden death unrelated to ventricular arrhythmias, which may not be treatable with defibrillation.[30] The results from these and other non-randomized analyses must be viewed with caution, because the observational/post hoc nature raises concern for confounding.

A study from the Get With the Guidelines program[31] highlights the uncertainty of when to implant these individuals. More than 13,000 patients with HHF were judged to be candidates for primary prevention ICDs. Of these patients, 19.0% had a previous ICD, 12.4% received an ICD during the index hospitalization, and 4.0% were discharged with a plan for outpatient implantation. Most (64.6%) were discharged without an ICD or a plan for outpatient implantation. Deferring the ICD leaves the patient unprotected from ventricular arrhythmias unless a wearable external defibrillator is used.

The effectiveness of ICD therapy to improve mortality revolves around the balance between the competing risks of arrhythmic death and non-arrhythmic death. In the absence of significant noncardiac comorbidities, the primary competing risk is heart failure death. From an SCD-HeFT (Sudden Cardiac Death in Heart Failure Trial) analysis,[32] relative mortality benefits seem to be dependent on baseline mortality risk. ICDs were associated with a 50% reduction in all-cause death in the lowest-risk patients (estimated annual mortality of 3%–5%), whereas no survival benefit was observed in the highest-risk patients (annual mortality >20%).

The risk of death 1 year after HHF exceeds 30%. No randomized trials have tested the efficacy of ICD implementation in the HHF setting. Further research is needed to improve patient selection and downstream effectiveness and efficiency of defibrillator therapy.[33] Future refinements in selection of ICD candidates must be shown to improve outcomes in prospective studies and move beyond LVEF to a multimodality approach. Risk stratification to determine which patients are at

Box 1
Priorities for electrophysiology research in HHF syndromes

- What is the optimal timing of ICD insertion surrounding an HHF?

- How can risk stratification be improved for sudden arrhythmic death at discharge after a HHF?

- Can novel biomarkers (such as ST2) identify patients at risk for sudden arrhythmic death?

- Does [123]I-*meta*-iodobenzylguanidine scintigraphy reliably identify patients at risk for sudden arrhythmic death at discharge?

- How can novel cardiac imaging modalities aid in patient selection for implantation of ICDs and CRT defibrillators and outcome prediction?

- What is the comparative efficacy of CRT defibrillators in patients with HHF relative to chronic heart failure with systolic dysfunction?

- Can biomarkers (such as galectin-3) help direct CRT candidates in patients who are hospitalized for heart failure?

- Does catheter ablation of atrial fibrillation have a role in the management of patients who are hospitalized for heart failure?

- What is the comparative efficacy of catheter ablation versus antiarrhythmic drug therapy for ventricular arrhythmias in patients who are hospitalized for heart failure?

- When and how should palliative care measures be implemented?

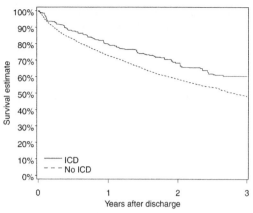

Fig. 3. Inverse probability-weighted survival for patients with heart failure with LVEF 35% or less. (*Reprinted from* Hernandez AF, Fonarow GC, Hammill BG, et al. Clinical effectiveness of implantable cardioverter-defibrillators among Medicare beneficiaries with heart failure. Circ Heart Fail 2010;3:10; with permission.)

low risk for early rehospitalization and death caused by progressive heart failure or other non-cardiac conditions may aid in the selection of patients as reasonable candidates for predischarge ICD implantation.

Serum ST2, a biomarker for cardiac strain, complements natriuretic peptide levels in predicting 1-year mortality in patients with HHF with both preserved and reduced LVEF.[34] In outpatients with chronic systolic heart failure, ST2 also predicts sudden cardiac death.[35] Novel imaging modalities, such as [123]I-*meta*-iodobenzylguanidine imaging, may also have a role in sudden death risk stratification before discharge.[36] These measures may have a role, alone or in conjunction with others, in determining the optimal time for ICD insertion in light of competing risks for nonarrhythmic death.

Cardiac Resynchronization Therapy

Cardiac resynchronization therapy (CRT) improves symptoms and survival in outpatients with chronic systolic heart failure and prolonged QRS duration. In general, its use is advocated only for persistent symptoms and not acute decompensation.[37] Background medications before CRT recommendation generally consist of angiotensin-converting enzyme inhibitors, angiotensin-receptor blockers, β-blockers, aldosterone antagonists, and diuretics.[14] Although New York Heart Association (NYHA) class is often used in CRT trials as an inclusion criterion, it may be more useful to think of CRT candidates as those with stage C heart failure.[38] All patients with HHF are, by definition, stage C or stage D.

A prolonged QRS duration is the accepted clinical criterion to assess cardiac dyssynchrony and potential candidacy for CRT. A prolonged QRS duration at the time of admission for heart failure has been established as highly associated with postdischarge mortality and morbidity.[39] Although the QRS duration during an exacerbation for heart failure is often the longest, most patients do not have significant changes during hospitalization.[39,40] CRT benefit is greatest in patients with a QRS duration of 150 ms or greater and a left bundle branch block pattern.[41,42]

A high degree of variability in CRT use exists in patients with HHF across hospitals in the United States.[43] De Sutter and colleagues[44] reported that only 25% of patients with HHF who were considered candidates for CRT were implanted during hospitalization or 6 months or less after discharge, despite electrophysiology consultation. Those implanted were younger and had fewer comorbid conditions. Another study compared CRT implantation between inpatients and elective outpatients.[45] Higher rates of comorbidities were also present in the inpatient group. Although inpatients had a higher risk of rehospitalization because of heart failure, this was no longer significant after adjustment for baseline characteristics. There was also no difference in the combined end point of all-cause mortality, decompensation requiring left ventricular assist device placement, and heart transplantation after adjustment. It is difficult to make inferences regarding the safety and outcomes of inpatient CRT implantation, because only successful CRT-implanted patients were included (ie, no control group without CRT). Inotropic-dependent patients are suboptimal candidates and have been excluded from CRT trials.[46]

In the absence of randomized studies in the population with HHF, the most reasonable course is to follow entry criteria from trials that have shown the benefit of CRT. In the CARE-HF (Cardiac Resynchronization in Heart Failure) trial,[47] patients waited a minimum of 6 weeks after a significant heart failure event before they could be considered for implantation. There is a critical need for clinical studies evaluating the role of biventricular pacing in patients with HHF. Outpatient trials of CRT have shown impressive reductions in hospitalizations. These and other benefits may be more pronounced in patients with HHF, in whom readmission rates approach 50%. Galectin-3 may some day assist in determining CRT candidacy, because a single level at the time of admission for heart failure predicts 4-year mortality and correlates with severity of heart failure in outpatient cohorts.[48,49]

Other areas of CRT investigation that may have relevance for patients with HHF include the use of imaging to assess potential candidates in the narrow QRS population and to optimize left ventricular lead position. Past investigation based on mechanical dyssynchrony in the absence of electrical dyssynchrony has been disappointing.[50,51] Imaging modalities assess changes in left ventricular mechanical synchrony, which is associated with response to CRT.[52] Novel imaging techniques, such as speckle tracking and phase analysis of gated single-photon emission computed tomography (SPECT), show promise and predict outcomes up to 1 year after implant.[53–55] Determination of the myocardial site of latest activation by phase analysis of gated SPECT may be valuable in the identification of patient-specific optimal position of the left ventricular lead.[56,57]

Pacemakers

Bradycardia resulting from sinus node dysfunction may lead to the development of heart failure.[58] Putative mechanisms include inadequate cardiac output, or increasing left ventricular volume and diastolic pressures.[59] Similar consequences may result from atrioventricular block. Because of a paucity of data, the optimal heart rate for patients with heart failure remains unknown. It is also uncertain whether the indications for non-CRT pacing in patients with heart failure could or should differ from the general population.

A study by Stecker and colleagues[60] suggested that atrial pacing to facilitate β-blocker use in those with resting sinus bradycardia is beneficial and cost-effective. In patients with resting heart rate of less than 68 beats per minute, mean survival was increased by 1.3 years in the pacemaker plus carvedilol group. Theoretically, patients with HHF with resting bradycardia that limits β-blocker therapy may have improved postdischarge outcomes with pacing and β-blocker therapy.

A high percentage of right ventricular pacing in patients with reduced LVEF may worsen heart failure, presumably because of the dyssynchronous activation of the paced ventricle. Decreasing the backup pacing rate or increasing the atrioventricular delay are options to maximize native conduction if right ventricular pacing is not obligatory.[61] Conversely, CRT should be programmed to achieve maximum biventricular pacing percentage. Device interrogation to meet these ends is reasonable in patients with HHF. A decrease in biventricular pacing may be caused by frequent premature ventricular complexes, lead dislodgement, atrial fibrillation, or enhanced native atrioventricular conduction.[62] Evidence is mounting for atrioventricular node ablation in patients with atrial fibrillation and CRT to achieve maximal biventricular pacing.[63]

Novel pacing modalities may hold promise in the ischemic population. In a pig model, localized high-frequency electric stimulation within the infarct zone may lead to favorable remodeling.[64] The mechanism is believed to be mediated through reduction of regional matrix metalloproteinase activity, and may some day be an option for patients with HHF refractory to current therapies. Vagal nerve stimulation has been shown in a rabbit model to have favorable effects on LVEF, most likely through suppression of acute inflammatory reactions.[65]

Catheter Ablation for Supraventricular Arrhythmias

In patients with atrial fibrillation, randomized clinical trials do not support superiority of a rhythm-control strategy over a rate-control strategy across a spectrum of patients with and without heart failure.[66–68] High crossover rates in clinical trials and limited efficacy of the available therapies preclude the definitive conclusion that maintaining sinus rhythm does not have benefit. Retrospective data suggest that patients who maintain sinus rhythm have better outcomes, irrespective of LVEF.[69,70] In outpatients with chronic heart failure, the noninferiority of a rhythm-control strategy may be a reflection of inadequate maintenance of sinus rhythm or adverse drug effects, rather than a lack of benefit of sinus rhythm per se.[71,72] The rate-control versus rhythm-control trials, including the Atrial Fibrillation in Congestive Heart Failure trial, did not include pulmonary vein isolation as a therapeutic option.[66–68]

Hsu and colleagues[73] evaluated pulmonary vein antral isolation in 58 consecutive patients with NYHA class II or greater symptoms and LVEF of less than 45%. Although these patients were not necessarily hospitalized at the time, 16% had at least 1 episode of class IV heart failure in the preceding 6 months and 3 patients were awaiting cardiac transplantation. After a mean follow-up of approximately 1 year, 78% remained in sinus rhythm. An absolute increase in the mean LVEF of 21% was believed to be caused by underlying tachycardia-induced cardiomyopathy. Patients with rapid atrial fibrillation and inadequate control using pharmacologic therapy may therefore be candidates for pulmonary vein isolation to prevent recurrent HHF admissions. Given the complexity of the procedure, return for an outpatient procedure is generally recommended.[74]

A rate-control strategy in patients with HHF has few data from systematic study.[75] For patients who are refractory to medical management, pacemaker implantation with ablation of the atrioventricular junction may be a reasonable option. If this approach is taken, those with reduced LVEF should be considered for CRT.[63,76,77] Selection of a conventional non-CRT pacemaker is recommended for those with preserved LVEF.[77]

Typical (cavotricuspid isthmus-dependent) atrial flutter is highly amenable to catheter ablation. Recurrence at 13 months was only 3.8% after cavotricuspid isthmus ablation compared with 29.5% in those treated with amiodarone in the LADIP (Loire-Ardéche-Drôme-Isére-Puy-de-Dôme) randomized trial.[78] Tachycardia-induced cardiomyopathy may occur in those with atrial flutter and reduced LVEF. Luchsinger and Steinberg reported an increase in mean LVEF from 30.9% to 41.3% in 11 patients who underwent cavotricuspid isthmus ablation for atrial flutter with rapid ventricular rate and LVEF less than 50%.[79] Patients with HHF exacerbated by atrial flutter may derive benefit from upfront ablation during hospitalization, but this hypothesis has not been systematically evaluated.

Supraventricular tachycardia traditionally encompasses atrioventricular nodal reentrant tachycardia, atrioventricular reentrant tachycardia, and atrial tachycardia. In the DIG (Digitalis Investigation Group) trial, these dysrrhythmias were a strong predictor for mortality and HHF, irrespective of LVEF.[80] Catheter ablation for regular supraventricular tachycardia has high success rates and low rates of adverse effects.[81–83] It is reasonable to proceed after clinical stabilization if the arrhythmia is a clear inciting factor that is refractory to medical management.

Catheter Ablation for Ventricular Arrhythmias

Ventricular tachycardia may cause hemodynamic compromise, ICD shocks, and worsening heart failure. Catheter ablation is effective in decreasing ventricular arrhythmias and ICD shocks; however, it is invasive, with potentially serious adverse effects.[84] Induction of unstable arrhythmias is often an integral part of the procedure. Routine ablation of ventricular tachycardia cannot be recommended during an HHF admission. Exceptions include incessant ventricular tachycardia or frequent ICD shocks.[74] For sustained arrhythmias, randomized data of catheter ablation versus antiarrhythmics requires investigation, and trials are ongoing.

Preliminary data suggest that ablation of frequent premature ventricular complexes in stable patients with heart failure may lead to normalization of LVEF.[85] The potential benefit is not immediate, so ablation in patients with HHF should not be routine practice but may be considered after outpatient stabilization. Targeting premature ventricular complexes that frequently trigger ventricular fibrillation may be considered in select patients.[86] Physicians should be cognizant of this situation, given that ICD shocks caused by ventricular fibrillation may worsen heart failure status.

Implantable Device Monitoring

Pacemakers, CRT devices, and ICDs have memory logs that may aid in assessing clinical status. Examples of some potentially available data include heart rates (both native and paced), frequency of atrial and ventricular pacing, mode switch episodes (both frequency and duration, which indicate atrial arrhythmias), and ventricular arrhythmia events (with or without shocks delivered). Some devices have more specialized data, such as intrathoracic impedance trends, heart rate variability, and patient activity trends. Theoretically, use of these data to identify dysrrhythmias that exacerbate heart failure status or early decompensation may avoid hospitalization, decrease the length of hospital stay, or prevent early readmission.

Mode switch episodes correlate with atrial fibrillation burden.[87] Rapid ventricular conduction during atrial fibrillation contributes to heart failure decompensation and represents an important therapeutic opportunity. Frequent shocks for both appropriate and inappropriate causes are associated with an increased risk of death; most commonly from progressive heart failure.[23] Review of intracardiac electrograms may be diagnostic. Interventions with antiarrhythmic medication, antitachycardia pacing algorithms, or catheter ablation may aid in decreasing episodes of ventricular tachycardia leading to ICD shocks.[84,88,89]

Decreases in intrathoracic impedance correlate with worsening congestion.[90] Intensive monitoring in the postdischarge period may aid optimization of inpatient and outpatient management and avoid rehospitalization. Unexpectedly, monitoring of intrathoracic impedance and other diagnostic parameters resulted in a 79% increase in readmissions for heart failure in the randomized DOT-HF (Diagnostic Outcome Trial in Heart Failure).[91]

Wireless pulmonary artery hemodynamic monitoring showed benefit in the population of outpatients with chronic heart failure with both reduced and preserved LVEF in the CHAMPION (Cardio-MEMS Heart Sensor Allows Monitoring of Pressure to Improve Outcomes in NYHA III HF Patients) trial.[92] Device use reduced admissions because of heart failure by 30%, improved quality-of-life parameters, and reduced mean length of stay in those with HHF within the preceding year.

Increased heart rate and decreased heart rate variability are linked to worse outcomes. Recently, an increased mean intrinsic heart rate measured via ICDs was associated with a higher rate of death or HHF.[93] Evaluation of mean heart rate in postdischarge visits may aid in titration of β-blockers to target heart rates.[94]

Many patients with heart failure have coexisting coronary artery disease.[95] In patients with an implantable device, the use of intracardiac electrogram monitoring to detect ST segment changes may facilitate timely diagnosis and treatment of acute coronary syndromes, thus avoiding further myocardial damage and preventing downstream hospitalization.[96]

Practical Considerations Before Implementation

Barriers may prevent implementation of therapies directed toward heart rhythm disorders in patients with HHF. First, there is a lack of randomized trials to support benefit in HHF syndromes. Without these data, there can be no mandate for interventions in the hospitalized setting. Even when patients are judged to be reasonable candidates and interventions have a high probability of enhancing treatment, other impediments may exist.

Patients are often under the care of internists or hospitalists who may have less familiarity with up-to-date, available treatments.[97] Conversely, patients who undergo systematic cardiac evaluation may have significant coronary artery disease, for which revascularization is recommended.[95] Current guidelines advocate delay in ICD or CRT consideration for up to 3 months to assess potential LVEF recovery. Longitudinal care should involve the patients' outpatient physicians, because they often know the medical and social situations the best. The transition from inpatient to outpatient care needs to have a plan to implement interventions that prevent rehospitalization and so they are not lost to follow-up.

Reimbursement structures with a bundled payment approach often create disincentives to provide nonpharmacologic electrophysiology-based interventions during HHF admissions. For example, a hospital and associated providers may be paid a fixed amount. The cost of catheter ablation, if performed during that hospitalization or soon after, may not be reimbursed. Thus, there becomes an incentive to discharge the patient with a plan for subsequent outpatient scheduling of the procedure at a later date. This practice may not be in the best interest of the patient. Recent studies on disease management programs for postdischarge heart failure have not integrated evaluation of nonpharmacologic electrophysiology-based interventions.[98]

Patients with congestion may be at a higher risk for procedural complications compared with euvolemic outpatients. The immediate effect of interventions implemented during HHF is not well studied. Examples of scenarios of particular concern include defibrillation threshold testing during ICD placement, intravenous contrast use during CRT implantation, and sudden rhythm changes during catheter ablation. Translation of these concerns into higher complication rates or worse outcomes has not been rigorously established. However, they are commonly cited as reasons not to proceed with interventions at the time of heart failure hospitalization.

Hospitalized patients may have higher rates of infection because of indwelling catheters, more virulent microorganisms in the hospital environment, physical deconditioning, and a generally higher susceptibility to infections. This finding is of particular concern for device implantation, because device infection is occasionally life-threatening and associated with prolonged antibiotic treatment and device explanation. Intervening while a patient has limited physical capability needs to be taken into context when considering invasive procedures.

Palliative Care

Palliative care is an important aspect of the care of patients with advanced heart failure.[99] Nonpharmacologic electrophysiology-based procedures have the potential to offer profound symptomatic or life-prolonging benefit, but may also lead to physical and mental distress. End of life is difficult to predict, even in very symptomatic individuals, so discussions regarding patient and family concerns should begin early. Specific issues that may arise include deactivation of therapies for tachyarrhythmias in implanted devices. For patients who opt for interventions, it is important to have a candid discussion of potential adverse events and the wishes of the patient and their family should they occur.

SUMMARY

HHF syndromes have high postdischarge mortality and morbidity. Few interventions during or soon after hospitalization improve long-term outcomes. Nonpharmacologic electrophysiology-based interventions have a significant impact on outpatients with chronic heart failure. The role of these therapies in patients with HHF is largely unknown because of lack of systematic investigation. The optimal timing of these interventions in the postdischarge period is not well defined. Studies to clarify mechanisms behind worsening heart failure and the potential roles of these electrophysiologic therapies are needed, given the poor outcomes.

DISCLOSURES

Dr Piccini has received grants for clinical research from Boston Scientific and Johnson & Johnson; is a consultant for Forest Laboratories, Johnson&Johnson, Medtronic, and Sanofi-Aventis. Dr Fonarowis a consultant for Novartis, Medtronic, and Gambro. Dr Knight receives fellowship support from Bard, Biosense Webster, Biotronik, Medtronic, and St Jude Medical; is a speaker for Biosense Webster, Biotronik, Boston Scientific, Medtronic, and St Jude Medical; is a consultant for Biosense Webster, Boston Scientific, and Cameron Health; and is an investigator for Biotronik, Cameron Health, Medtronic, and St Jude Medical. Dr Butler is an investigator for Medtronic, Boston Scientific, and GE Healthcare. Dr Gheorghiade is a consultant for Abbott Laboratories, Astellas, AstraZeneca, Bayer Schering Pharma, CorThera, Cytokinetics Inc, Debio-Pharm, Errekappa Therapeuitici, GlaxoSmith-Kline, Johnson & Johnson, Medtronic, Merck, Novartis Pharma, Otsuka Pharmaceuticals, Pericor Therapeutics, Protein Design Laboratories, Sanofi-Aventis, Sigma Tau, and Solvay Pharmaceuticals. All other authors have reported that they have no relationships to disclose relevant to the contents of this article.

REFERENCES

1. Braunwald E. Cardiovascular medicine at the turn of the millennium: triumphs, concerns, and opportunities. N Engl J Med 1997;337:1360–9.
2. Roger VL, Go AS, Lloyd-Jones DM, et al. Heart disease and stroke statistics–2012 update: a report from the American Heart Association. Circulation 2012;125:e2–220.
3. Haldeman GA, Croft JB, Giles WH, et al. Hospitalization of patients with heart failure: National Hospital Discharge Survey, 1985 to 1995. Am Heart J 1999;137:352–60.
4. Jencks SF, Williams MV, Coleman EA. Rehospitalizations among patients in the Medicare fee-for-service program. N Engl J Med 2009;360: 1418–28.
5. Gheorghiade M, Zannad F, Sopko G, et al. Acute heart failure syndromes: current state and framework for future research. Circulation 2005;112: 3958–68.
6. Ahmed A, Allmann RM, Fonarow GC, et al. Incident heart failure hospitalization and subsequent mortality in chronic heart failure: a propensity-matched study. J Card Fail 2008;14:211–8.
7. Fonarow GC, Albert NM, Curtis AB, et al. Improving evidence-based care for heart failure in outpatient cardiology practices: primary results of the registry to improve the use of evidence-based heart failure therapies in the outpatient setting (IMPROVE HF). Circulation 2010;122:585–96.
8. Fonarow GC, Abraham WT, Albert NM, et al. Influence of beta-blocker continuation or withdrawal on outcomes in patients hospitalized with heart failure: findings from the OPTIMIZE-HF program. J Am Coll Cardiol 2008;52:190–9.
9. Hamaguchi S, Kinugawa S, Tsuchihashi-Makaya M, et al. Spironolactone use at discharge was associated with improved survival in hospitalized patients with systolic heart failure. Am Heart J 2010;160:1156–62.
10. Rathore SS, Masoudi FA, Wang Y, et al. Socioeconomic status, treatment, and outcomes among elderly patients hospitalized with heart

failure: findings from the National Heart Failure Project. Am Heart J 2006;152:371–8.

11. Curtis LH, Greiner MA, Hammill BG, et al. Early and long-term outcomes of heart failure in elderly persons, 2001-2005. Arch Intern Med 2008;168:2481–8.

12. Jessup M, Abraham WT, Casey DE, et al, on behalf of the 2005 Guideline Update for the Diagnosis and Management of Chronic Heart Failure in the Adult Writing Committee. 2009 focused update: ACCF/AHA guidelines for the diagnosis and management of heart failure in adults: a report of the American College of Cardiology/American Heart Association Task Force on Practice Guidelines. J Am Coll Cardiol 2009;53:1343–82.

13. Dickstein K, Vardas PE, Auricchio A, et al. 2010 focused update of ESC guidelines on device therapy in heart failure: an update of the 2008 ESC guidelines for the diagnosis and treatment of acute and chronic heart failure and the 2007 USC guidelines for cardiac and resynchronization therapy. Eur Heart J 2010;31:2677–87.

14. Stevenson WG, Hernandez AF, Carson PE, et al. Indications for cardiac resynchronization therapy: 2011 update from the Heart Failure Society of America guideline committee. J Card Fail 2012; 18:94–106.

15. Fonarow GC, Albert NM, Curtis AB, et al. Associations between outpatient heart failure process-of-care measures and mortality. Circulation 2011; 123:1601–10.

16. McMurray JJ, Adamopoulos S, Anker SD, et al. ESC guidelines for the diagnosis and treatment of acute and chronic heart failure: The Task Force for the Diagnosis and Treatment of Acute and Chronic Heart Failure 2012 of the European Society of Cardiology. Developed in collaboration with the Heart Failure Association (HFA) of the ESC. Eur Heart J 2012;33:1787–847.

17. Solomon SD, Dobson J, Pocock S, et al. Influence of nonfatal hospitalization for heart failure on subsequent mortality in patients with chronic heart failure. Circulation 2007;116:1482–7.

18. Gheorghiade M, Pang PS. Acute heart failure syndromes. J Am Coll Cardiol 2009;53:557–73.

19. Myerburg RJ, Reddy V, Castellanos A. Indications for implantable cardioverter-defibrillators based on evidence and judgment. J Am Coll Cardiol 2009;54:747–63.

20. Moss AJ, Zareba W, Hall WJ, et al. Prophylactic implantation of a defibrillator in patients with myocardial infarction and reduced ejection fraction. N Engl J Med 2002;346:877–83.

21. Bardy GH, Lee KL, Poole JE, et al. Amiodarone or an implantable cardioverter-defibrillator for congestive heart failure. N Engl J Med 2005;352:225–37.

22. Goldenberg I, Moss AJ, Hall WJ, et al. Causes and consequences of heart failure after prophylactic implantation of a defibrillator in the Multicenter Automatic Defibrillator Implantation Trial II. Circulation 2006;113:2810–7.

23. Poole JE, Johnson GW, Hellkamp AS, et al. Prognostic importance of defibrillator shocks in patients with heart failure. N Engl J Med 2008;359: 1009–17.

24. Ellenbogun KA, Levine JH, Berger RD, et al. Are implantable cardioverter defibrillator shocks a surrogate for sudden cardiac death in patients with nonischemic cardiomyopathy? Circulation 2006; 113:776–82.

25. Dhar R, Alsheikh-Ali AA, Estes NA 3rd, et al. Association of prolonged QRS duration with ventricular tachyarrhythmias and sudden cardiac death in the Multicenter Automatic Defibrillator Implantation Trial II (MADIT-II). Heart Rhythm 2009;5: 807–13.

26. The DAVID Trial Investigators. Dual-chamber pacing or ventricular backup pacing in patients with an implantable defibrillator. JAMA 2002; 288:3115–23.

27. Stevenson LW, Desai AS. Selecting patients for discussion of the ICD as primary prevention for sudden death in heart failure. J Card Fail 2006;12: 407–12.

28. Hernandez AF, Fonarow GC, Hammill BG, et al. Clinical effectiveness of implantable cardioverter-defibrillators among Medicare beneficiaries with heart failure. Circ Heart Fail 2010;3:7–13.

29. Wang NC, Piccini JP, Konstam MA, et al. Implantable cardioverter-defibrillators in patients hospitalized for heart failure with chronically reduced left ventricular ejection fraction. Am J Ther 2010;17: e78–87.

30. Mitchell LB, Pineda EA, Titus JL, et al. Sudden death in patients with implantable cardioverter defibrillators. J Am Coll Cardiol 2002;39:1323–8.

31. Hernandez AF, Fonarow GC, Liang L, et al. Sex and racial differences in the use of implantable cardioverter-defibrillators among patients hospitalized with heart failure. JAMA 2007;298:1525–32.

32. Levy WC, Lee KL, Hellkamp AS, et al. Maximizing survival benefit with primary prevention implantable cardioverter-defibrillator therapy in a heart failure population. Circulation 2009;120:835–42.

33. Tung R, Zimetbaum P, Josephson ME. A critical appraisal of implantable cardioverter-defibrillator therapy for the prevention of sudden cardiac death. J Am Coll Cardiol 2008;52(14):1111–21.

34. Rehman SU, Mueller T, Januzzi JL Jr. Characteristics of the novel interleukin family biomarker ST2 in patients with acute heart failure. J Am Coll Cardiol 2008;52:1458–65.

35. Pascual-Figal DA, Ordoñez-Llanos J, Tornel PL, et al. Soluble ST2 for predicting sudden cardiac death in patients with chronic heart failure and

left ventricular systolic dysfunction. J Am Coll Cardiol 2009;54(23):2174–9.

36. Carrió I, Cowie MR, Yamazaki J, et al. Cardiac sympathetic imaging with mIBG in heart failure. JACC Cardiovasc Imaging 2010;3:92–100.

37. Ujeyl A, Stevenson LW. Populations for CRT devices. Heart Rhythm 2009;6:1373–7.

38. Jessup M. MADIT-CRT–breathtaking or time to catch our breath? N Engl J Med 2009;361:1394–6.

39. Wang NC, Maggioni AP, Konstam MA, et al. Clinical implications of QRS duration in patients hospitalized with worsening heart failure and reduced left ventricular ejection fraction. JAMA 2008;299:2656–66.

40. Aranda JM Jr, Carlson ER, Pauly DF, et al. QRS duration variability in patients with heart failure. Am J Cardiol 2002;90:335–7.

41. Stavrakis S, Lazzara R, Thadani U. The benefit of cardiac resynchonization therapy and QRS duration: a meta-analysis. J Cardiovasc Electrophysiol 2012;23:163–8.

42. Zareba W, Klein H, Cygankiewicz I, et al. Effectiveness of cardiac resynchronization therapy by QRS morphology in the Multicenter Automatic Defibrillator Implantation Trial–Cardiac Resynchronization Therapy (MADIT-CRT). Circulation 2011;123:1061–72.

43. Piccini JP, Hernandez AF, Dai D, et al. Use of cardiac resynchronization therapy in patients hospitalized with heart failure. Circulation 2008;118:926–33.

44. De Sutter J, Weytjens C, Van de Veire N, et al. Prevalence of potential cardiac resynchronization therapy candidates and actual use of cardiac resynchronization therapy in patients hospitalized for heart failure. Eur J Heart Fail 2011;13:412–5.

45. Ajijola OA, Macklin EA, Moore SA, et al. Inpatient vs. elective outpatient cardiac resynchronization therapy device implantation and long-term clinical outcome. Europace 2010;12:1745–9.

46. Bhattacharya S, Abebe K, Simon M, et al. Role of cardiac resynchronization in end-stage heart failure patients requiring inotrope therapy. J Card Fail 2010;16(12):931–7.

47. Cleland JG, Daubert JC, Erdmann E, et al. The effect of cardiac resynchronization on morbidity and mortality in heart failure. N Engl J Med 2005;352:1539–49.

48. Shah RV, Chen-Tournoux AA, Picard MH, et al. Galectin-3, cardiac structure and function, and long-term mortality in patients with acutely decompensated heart failure. Eur J Heart Fail 2010;12:826–32.

49. Felker GM, Fiuzat M, Shaw LK, et al. Galectin-3 in ambulatory patients with heart failure: results from the HF-ACTION study. Circ Heart Fail 2012;5:72–8.

50. Beshai JF, Grimm RA, Nagueh S, et al. Cardiac-resynchronization therapy in heart failure with narrow QRS complexes. N Engl J Med 2007;357:2461–71.

51. Chung ES, Leon AR, Tavazzi L, et al. Results of the predictors of response to CRT (PROSPECT) trial. Circulation 2008;117:2608–16.

52. Bax JJ, Marwick TH, Molhoek SG, et al. Left ventricular dyssynchrony predicts benefit of cardiac resynchronization therapy in patients with end-stage heart failure before pacemaker implantation. Am J Cardiol 2003;92:1238–40.

53. Friehling M, Chen J, Saba S, et al. A prospective pilot study to evaluate the relationship between acute change in left ventricular synchrony after cardiac resynchronization therapy and patient outcome using a single-injection gated SPECT protocol. Circ Cardiovasc Imaging 2011;4:532–9.

54. Aljaroudi WA, Hage FG, Hermann D, et al. Relation of left-ventricular dyssynchrony by phase analysis of gated SPECT images and cardiovascular events in patients with implantable cardiac defibrillators. J Nucl Cardiol 2010;17:398–404.

55. Lim P, Donal E, Lafitte S, et al. Muticentre study using strain delay index for predicting response to cardiac resynchronization therapy (MUSIC study). Eur J Heart Fail 2011;13:984–91.

56. Boogers MJ, Chen J, van Bommel RJ, et al. Optimal left ventricular lead position assessed with phase analysis on gated myocardial perfusion SPECT. Eur J Nucl Med Mol Imaging 2011;38(2):230–8.

57. Cavallino C, Rondano E, Magnani A, et al. Baseline asynchrony, assessed circumferentially using temporal uniformity of strain, besides coincidence between site of latest mechanical activation and presumed left ventricular lead position, predicts favourable prognosis after resynchronization therapy. Int J Cardiovasc Imaging 2012;28:1011–21.

58. Alboni P, Menozzi C, Brignole M, et al. Effects of permanent pacemaker and oral theophylline in sick sinus syndrome. The THEOPACE study: a randomized controlled trial. Circulation 1997;96:260–6.

59. Alboni P, Brignole M, Menozzi C, et al. Is sinus bradycardia a factor facilitating overt heart failure? Eur Heart J 1999;20:252–5.

60. Stecker EC, Fendrick AM, Knight BP, et al. Prophylactic pacemaker use to allow β-blocker therapy in patients with chronic heart failure with bradycardia. Am Heart J 2006;151:820–8.

61. Sweeney MO, Prinzen FW. A new paradigm for physiologic ventricular pacing. J Am Coll Cardiol 2006;47:282–8.

62. Koplan BA, Kalpan AJ, Weiner S, et al. Heart failure decompensation and all-cause mortality in relation to percent biventricular pacing in patients with

heart failure: is a goal of 100% biventricular pacing necessary. J Am Coll Cardiol 2009;53:355–60.

63. Ganesan AN, Brooks AG, Roberts-Thomson KC, et al. Role of AV nodal ablation in cardiac resynchronization in patients with coexistent atrial fibrillation and heart failure: a systematic review. J Am Coll Cardiol 2012;59:719–25.

64. Murherjee R, Rivers WT, Ruddy JM, et al. Long-term localized high-frequency electric stimulation within the myocardial infarct: effects on matrix metalloproteinases and regional remodeling. Circulation 2010;122:20–32.

65. Uemura K, Zheng C, Li M, et al. Early short-term vagal nerve stimulation attenuates cardiac remodeling after reperfused myocardial infarction. J Card Fail 2010;16:689–99.

66. The AFFIRM Investigators. A comparison of rate control and rhythm control in patients with atrial fibrillation. N Engl J Med 2002;437:1825–33.

67. Van Gelder IC, Hagens VE, Bosker HA, et al. A comparison of rate control and rhythm control in patients with recurrent persistent atrial fibrillation. N Engl J Med 2002;347:1834–40.

68. Roy D, Talajic M, Nattel S, et al. Rhythm control versus rate control for atrial fibrillation and heart failure. N Engl J Med 2008;358:2667–77.

69. Pedersen OD, Bagger H, Keller N, et al. Efficacy of dofetilide in the treatment of atrial fibrillation-flutter in patients with reduced left ventricular function: a Danish Investigations of Arrhythmia and Mortality ON Dofetilide (DIAMOND) Substudy. Circulation 2001;104:292–6.

70. Olsson LG, Swedberg K, Ducharme A, et al. Atrial fibrillation and risk of clinical events in chronic heart failure with and without left ventricular systolic dysfunction. Results from the Candesartan in Heart failure-Assessment of Reduction in Mortality and morbidity (CHARM) Program. J Am Coll Cardiol 2006;47:1997–2004.

71. Lafuente-Lafuente C, Mouly S, Longâs-Tejero M, et al. Antiarrhythmic drugs for maintaining sinus rhythm after cardioversion of atrial fibrillation: a systematic review of randomized controlled trials. Arch Intern Med 2006;166:719–28.

72. Saksena S, Slee A, Waldo AL, et al. Cardiovascular outcomes in the AFFIRM trial (Atrial Fibrillation Follow-Up Investigation of Rhythm Management): an assessment of individual antiarrhythmic drug therapies compared with rate control with propensity score-matched analyses. J Am Coll Cardiol 2011;58:1975–85.

73. Hsu LF, Jaïs P, Sanders P, et al. Catheter ablation for atrial fibrillation in congestive heart failure. N Engl J Med 2004;351:2373–83.

74. Knight BP, Jacobson JT. Assessing patients for catheter ablation during hospitalization for acute heart failure. Heart Fail Rev 2011;16:467–76.

75. DiMarco JP. Atrial fibrillation and acute decompensated heart failure. Circ Heart Fail 2009;2:72–3.

76. Doshi RN, Daoud EG, Fellows C, et al. Left ventricular-based cardiac stimulation Post AV nodal ablation Evaluation (The PAVE Study). J Cardiovasc Electrophysiol 2005;16:1160–5.

77. Epstein AE, DiMarco JP, Ellenbogun KA, et al. ACC/AHA/HRS 2008 guidelines for device-based therapy of cardiac rhythm abnormalities: a report of the American College of Cardiology/American Heart Association Task Force on Practice Guidelines (Writing Committee to Revise the ACC/AHA/NASPE 2002 Guideline Update for Implantation of Cardiac Pacemakers and Antiarrhythmia Devices). J Am Coll Cardiol 2008;51:e1–62.

78. Da Costa A, Thévenin J, Roche F, et al. Results from the Loire-Ardéche-Drôme-Isére-Puy-de-Dôme (LADIP) trial on atrial flutter, a multicentric prospective randomized study comparing amiodarone and radiofrequency ablation after the first episode of symptomatic atrial flutter. Circulation 2006;114:1676–81.

79. Luchsinger JA, Steinberg JA. Resolution of cardiomyopathy after ablation for atrial flutter. J Am Coll Cardiol 1998;32:205–10.

80. Mathew J, Hunsberger S, Fleg J, et al. Incidence, predictive factors, and prognostic significant of supraventricular tachyarrhythmias in congestive heart failure. Chest 2000;118:914–22.

81. Jackman WM, Beckman KJ, McClelland JH, et al. Treatment of supraventricular tachycardia due to atrioventricular nodal reentry by radiofrequency catheter ablation of slow-pathway conduction. N Engl J Med 1992;327:313–8.

82. Jackman WM, Wang X, Friday KJ, et al. Catheter ablation of accessory atrioventricular pathways (Wolff-Parkinson-White syndrome) by radiofrequency current. N Engl J Med 1991;324:1605–11.

83. Kay GN, Chong F, Epstein AE, et al. Radiofrequency ablation for treatment of primary atrial tachycardias. J Am Coll Cardiol 1993;21:901–9.

84. Reddy VK, Reynolds MR, Neuzil P, et al. Prophylactic catheter ablation for the prevention of defibrillator therapy. N Engl J Med 2007;357:2657–65.

85. Bogun F, Crawford T, Reich S, et al. Radiofrequency ablation of frequent, idiopathic premature ventricular complexes: comparison with a control group without intervention. Heart Rhythm 2006;4:863–7.

86. Marrouche NF, Verma A, Wazni O, et al. Mode of initiation and ablation of ventricular fibrillation storms in patients with ischemic cardiomyopathy. J Am Coll Cardiol 2004;43:1715–20.

87. Passman RS, Weinberg KM, Freher M, et al. Accuracy of mode switch algorithms for detection of atrial tachyarrhythmias. J Cardiovasc Electrophysiol 2004;15:773–7.

88. Connolly SJ, Dorian P, Roberts RS, et al. Comparison of β-blockers, amiodarone, plus β-blockers, or sotalol for prevention of shocks from implantable cardioverter defibrillators. JAMA 2006;295:165–71.

89. Larsen GK, Evans J, Lambert WE, et al. Shock burden and increased mortality in implantable cardioverter-defibrillator patients. Heart Rhythm 2011;8:1881–6.

90. Yu CM, Wang L, Chau E, et al. Intrathoracic impedance monitoring in patients with heart failure: correlation with fluid status and feasibility of early warning preceding hospitalization. Circulation 2005;112:841–8.

91. van Veldhuisen DJ, Braunschweig F, Conraads V, et al. Intrathoracic impedance monitoring, audible patient alerts, and outcome in patients with heart failure. Circulation 2011;124:1719–26.

92. Abraham WT, Adamson PB, Bourge RC, et al. Wireless pulmonary artery haemodynamic monitoring in chronic heart failure: a randomized controlled trial. Lancet 2011;377:658–66.

93. Ahmadi-Kashani M, Kessler DJ, Day J, et al. Heart rate predicts outcomes in an implantable cardioverter-defibrillator population. Circulation 2009;120:2040–5.

94. Hall AS, Palmer S. The heart rate hypothesis: ready to be tested. Heart 2008;94:561–5.

95. Flaherty JD, Bax JJ, De Luca L, et al. Acute heart failure syndromes in patients with coronary artery disease: early assessment and treatment. J Am Coll Cardiol 2009;53:254–63.

96. Fischell TA, Fischell DR, Avezum A, et al. Initial clinical results using intracardiac electrogram monitoring to detect and alert patients during coronary plaque rupture and ischemia. J Am Coll Cardiol 2010;56:1089–98.

97. Bellotti P, Badano LP, Acquarone N, et al. Specialty-related differences in the epidemiology, clinical profile, management and outcome of patients hospitalized for heart failure. Eur Heart J 2001;22:596–604.

98. Eapen ZJ, Reed SD, Curtis LH, et al. Do heart failure disease management programs make financial sense under a bundled payment system? Am Heart J 2011;161:916–22.

99. Goodlin SJ. Palliative care in congestive heart failure. J Am Coll Cardiol 2009;54:386–96.

The Role of Micronutrients and Macronutrients in Patients Hospitalized for Heart Failure

Tobias D. Trippel[a], Stefan D. Anker, MD, PhD[b,c],
Stephan von Haehling, MD, PhD[c],*

KEYWORDS

- Nutrition • Heart failure • Metabolism • Micronutrients • Wasting • Sarcopenia

KEY POINTS

- Nutritional surveys and observational studies indicate that deficiencies in micronutrients and macronutrients may complicate the clinical syndrome of heart failure (HF).
- Patients at risk for wasting or who present with clinical manifestations such as cachexia or muscle wasting are especially prone to nutritional deficiencies.
- The current understanding of the detrimental pathophysiology of HF leaves room for suggestive metabolomic concepts that include supplementation of micronutrients and macronutrients in these patients.
- Myocardial energetics and nutrient metabolism represent potential treatment targets in HF.
- Lipids, proteins, and carbohydrates along with vitamins, amino acids, and other trace elements are under evaluation in this setting.
- Supplementation of ferric carboxymaltose has recently been identified to improve iron status, functional capacity, and quality of life in patients with HF.
- Further interventional studies investigating the role of micronutrients and macronutrients are needed to close the gap in evidence regarding patients with HF.

INTRODUCTION

Heart failure (HF) is a chronic progressive disease with a debilitating impact on the individual patient's life. Approximately 5.5 million patients in the United States suffer from HF, and more than 550,000 patients are diagnosed with HF for the first time each year.[1] The prevalence of symptomatic HF is estimated to range from 0.4% to 2.0% in the general European population,[2] putting HF among the most important causes of morbidity and mortality in industrialized societies.[3] Approximately 14 million patients have been diagnosed with HF in the European Union alone.[3]

Conflict of interest: Tobias D. Trippel has nothing to disclose; Stefan D. Anker has served as a paid consultant and/or has received research grants from Professional Dietetics, Fresenius Medical Care, GSK, Helsinn, Lilly Inc, Amgen, Psioxus, Bosch, and Solartium Dietetics; Stephan von Haehling has served as a paid consultant for Pfizer, Professional Dietetics, and Solartium Dietetics.

[a] Department of Cardiology, Campus Virchow Klinikum, Charité – Universitätsmedizin Berlin, Augustenburger Platz 1, Berlin D-13353, Germany; [b] IRCCS San Raffaele, Center for Clinical and Basic Research, 00166, Rome, Italy; [c] Applied Cachexia Research, Department of Cardiology, Campus Virchow Klinikum, Charité – Universitätsmedizin Berlin, Augustenburger Platz 1, Berlin D-13353, Germany
* Corresponding author. Applied Cachexia Research, Medizinische Klinik mit Schwerpunkt Kardiologie, Campus Virchow Klinikum, Charité – Universitätsmedizin Berlin, Augustenburger Platz 1, Berlin D-13353, Germany.
E-mail address: stephan.von.haehling@web.de

Heart Failure Clin 9 (2013) 345–357
http://dx.doi.org/10.1016/j.hfc.2013.05.001
1551-7136/13/$ – see front matter © 2013 Elsevier Inc. All rights reserved.

Despite standardized care[4] and adjusted medical therapy,[3] the prognosis of patients hospitalized for HF rivals that of highly malignant cancers.[5] Similar to metastatic disease, HF often leads to undernourishment and wasting, which are independent risk factors for mortality in these patients.[6,7] Consequently, the evaluation of body composition[8] as well as the nutritional assessment and support[9] of hospitalized patients with HF are of high clinical relevance to medical caregivers. Having identified the clinical problem, the question remains: how to tackle it? And is there a role for the enteral or parenteral supplementation of micronutrients and macronutrients in these patients?

WASTING, CACHEXIA, AND SARCOPENIA

Physicians have observed wasting in many chronic illnesses, including

- Cancer
- Sepsis
- Chronic kidney disease
- Chronic obstructive pulmonary disease
- AIDS

Often, the development of cachexia unveils the terminal stages of these disorders, usually carrying a devastating prognosis with it. Increased mortality was reported for patients suffering from cardiac cachexia,[6] a complex syndrome that affects multiple body systems[10] and that has only limited treatment options.

Over the past decade, numerous studies have investigated the association of anabolic/catabolic imbalance, adaptive changes in inflammatory and neurohormonal activation, malnutrition, malabsorption, metabolic dysfunction, and apoptosis in the pathogenesis of wasting in HF.[11] Knowledge of the mechanistic cornerstones of cachexia has considerably improved, and some potential treatment targets have been identified.[12] Rather than discussing the intricate catabolic process in patients with HF as a generalized wasting process, a specific approach to different physiologic systems, balance of micronutrients and macronutrients, and body composition has emerged in the field.

Patients with chronic HF have better survival with higher rather than normal body mass index (BMI). However, all measurements need to be made in an edema-free status, which is not usually available during times of hospitalization. The phenomenon of this supposedly protective effect of obesity in chronic illness is known as the obesity paradox.[13] Yet, BMI alone has been shown to be only an insufficient indicator of true nutritional status in patients with HF.[14] More detailed approaches to the analysis of nutritional status and body composition have been undertaken to look at the specific loss of muscle, fat, and bone mass or lack of plasma proteins.

Recent advances in the understanding of the pathophysiology of peripheral muscle wasting in cardiac cachexia have led to incremental interest in the role of sarcopenia in HF[15,16] as a possible indicator of frailty and a poor prognosis. Sarcopenia is a term that describes the process of losing muscle mass and muscle strength with advancing age, and a debate exists whether or not the term should be extended to loss of muscle mass and function in chronic illness as well.[17,18] In general, the term describes loss of appendicular skeletal muscle mass that exceeds two standard deviations (SDs) of a healthy, young population. Some investigators also consider functional parameters such as gait speed for the diagnosis of sarcopenia.[19]

Fülster and colleagues[20] have identified muscle wasting in 39 (19.5%) of 200 prospectively enrolled patients with chronic HF, a substudy of the Studies Investigating Co-morbidities Aggravating HF (SICA-HF) study,[21] which is ongoing. Sarcopenia was associated with reduced muscle strength, lower total peak oxygen consumption (peak V_{O_2} [oxygen consumption], 1173 ± 433 vs 1622 ± 456 mL/min), and more advanced disease in this study, indicating a reduction of functional capacity beyond cardiac impairment alone. Because patients with lower muscle mass are known to be at greater risk for falls and immobilization, these findings may impose great socioeconomic impact as well. Sarcopenia therefore represents an important aspect of a cascade of decay not only in elderly patients with HF and makes it an interesting treatment target. It is not known whether or not muscle wasting per se plays a role in hospitalization rates of patients with HF or whether it increases the length of hospital stay; however, it seems that nutritional supplementation may be worthwhile to support muscle function and strength, for example by use of essential amino acids.[22–24]

MALNUTRITION

In daily clinical practice, relevant malnutrition has been established in 20% to 70% of patients with HF[25–27] and is believed to further complicate this clinical syndrome. It affects ambulatory as well as hospitalized patients and may especially add insult to injury in patients at greater risk of wasting, or in patients who present already with clinical manifestations such as cachexia or sarcopenia.

The state of malnutrition is not limited to an inadequate diet. Anorexia, the state of reduced appetite and food intake, is a common trigger of malnourishment in these patients.[28,29] Precipitating factors can be

- Psychosocial (clinical depression, reduced self-care behavior, or social isolation)
- Aging and disease related (the decline of olfactory and gustatory food appreciation, nausea, and early satiety from congestive hepatopathy and gastropathy)
- Iatrogenic (polypharmacy, calorie and salt restriction, and weight management).[29]

However, it is not merely the anorectic deposition that should be blamed as the singular underlying reason for malnutrition in this population.[28]

Inadequate Absorption of Nutrients

Disturbed intestinal microcirculation with decreased gut energy supply and intestinal ischemia may alter the intestinal function and not allow for adequate absorption of micronutrients and macronutrients. Abdominal and gut edema with dysfunctional intestinal barriers[30] and consequently increased permeability, exposure to endotoxins, and chronic inflammation may impair mucosa function, nutrient uptake,[31] and even foster protein loss.[32] In a study by Arutyunov and colleagues,[33] loss of nutrients was highest in cachectic patients with HF, with up to 24% loss of fat and 19% loss of protein via stool, compared with 20% and 16%, respectively, in patients with New York Heart Association (NYHA) functional class III and IV without cachexia (both $P<.05$). A reduction by 54% of active and by 34% of passive carrier-mediated intestinal transport was observed in 20 patients with HF (12 edematous and 8 non-edematous) compared with 8 healthy controls ($P<.0001$) by Sandek and colleagues.[34] This reduced integrity of mucosal transporters is likely to contribute significantly to a wide range of nutrient deficiency, causing malnutrition and further fueling the wasting process.

Medication-Mediated Nutritive Imbalances

The therapy recommended by guidelines[3,4] for patients suffering from HF includes

- Angiotensin-converting enzyme inhibitors (ACEi)
- Angiotensin receptor blockers (ARB)
- Aldosterone antagonists (MRA)
- β-blockers (BB)

These potentially life-prolonging ACEi, ARB, MRA, and BB can lead to electrolyte abnormalities, especially hyperkalemia and zinc deficiency,

and predispose to some vitamin and micronutrient deficits.[35,36] Because decongestion is considered the mainstay of symptomatic HF therapy, thiazide-type and loop diuretics are frequently prescribed in this population.[37] It is self-evident that not only aggressive diuresis in acutely decompensated patients with HF but also routine titration of diuretics in the ambulatory setting are often driven by clinical signs and symptoms of HF.

Yue[38] determined difference of thiamine diphosphate serum levels in 99 patients admitted to the emergency department. In this cross-sectional analysis of 81 patients suffering from HF who received furosemide treatment and in 18 patients suffering from acute myocardial infarction without signs and symptoms of HF who did not receive any loop diuretics, no significant difference was found in thiamine diphosphate levels.

Härdig[39] performed a cross-sectional measurement of thiamine, thiamine phosphate, and thiamine diphosphate concentrations in 41 patients hospitalized for HF and 34 ambulatory elderly individuals without HF. No difference was found in thiamine and thiamine diphosphate levels. However, these investigators identified a difference in thiamine phosphate levels, indicating a possibly altered thiamine metabolism.

Suter[40] concluded that older hospitalized patients are at increased risk for thiamine deficiency when treated with furosemide. It becomes clear that the constant temptation of rapid symptom relief is complicated by possibly severe side effects of electrolyte imbalances or vitamin excretion such as loss of potassium, magnesium, or calcium and B vitamins[41] (a process accelerated when combining thiazide and loop diuretics[42] to achieve sequential nephron blockade).

Hypercatabolism

Patients with HF frequently suffer from chronic inflammatory processes and increased sympathetic activity, which are documented by persistently high levels of circulating inflammatory cytokines and catecholamines. Some patients are further characterized by resting hypermetabolism[43] and increased protein breakdown, in which anabolic and catabolic hormones may play a crucial role.[44] Cardiopulmonary decompensation with acute hospitalization or strenous stays in the intensive care unit may then further contribute to hypercatabolism, and increase the consumption of antioxidant nutrients as a result of increased oxidative stress.[45] Antiinflammatory and nutritional interventions[46] have been discussed as limiting this clinical hypercatabolism and a catabolism-mediated increased prevalence of malnutrition in these patients.[47]

Changed Metabolism and Energetics

Micronutrients and macronutrients are the foundation of any metabolic system. Metabolomics has enhanced our understanding of myocardial metabolism and energetics[48] and assists our understanding of the larger metabolic derangements that accompany myocardial dysfunction.

An increased use of carbohydrates as preferred substrates for metabolism and adenosine triphosphate (ATP) generation is seen in some patients with HF. Although noncarbohydrate substrates such as fatty acids provide the highest energy yield per molecule of metabolized substrate, carbohydrates such as glucose provide greater efficiency in producing high-energy products per oxygen consumed.[49] Consequently, inherent alterations in the mitochondrial electron transport chain, ATP production, a relative change in oxygen usage, and efficiency may occur. Ardehali and colleagues[50] propose cardiac energetics, represented by the myocardial substrate metabolism, to be considered as a potential target for therapy in HF. Going beyond myocardial metabolism alone, several attempts at nuclear magnetic resonance–based metabolite pattern recognition have been made to capture the organism-wide metabolomic impact that HF puts on these patients. The rationale of this metabolomic profiling and search for specific substrate signatures is (1) the identification of pathophysiologic mechanisms,[51] (2) hypothesis generation for new therapeutic options, and (3) identification of novel biomarkers for diagnosis, therapy monitoring, and prognosis. A better understanding of the dynamic shift in energy substrate use and metabolism may enhance our understanding of special nutritive needs in these patients and nurture therapeutic options. For the reasons mentioned earlier, an adequate supply of micronutrients and macronutrients should not be taken for granted in the population with HF, particularly not during times of intensive stress such as periods of hospitalization with or without decompensation.

MACRONUTRIENTS
Fat

As discussed earlier, fatty acids are the preferred metabolic substrates of the healthy heart to generate energy.[52] Nutritional fat, as a macronutrient used for cardiac energetics, can be categorized into saturated and unsaturated fatty acids (UFAs). UFAs are either mono-UFAs or poly-UFAs, and in addition, UFAs can be further divided

into cis-UFAs, which are the most common in nature and are believed to be beneficial, and trans-UFAs, which are found in margarine and vegetable oils, but are rare in unprocessed food. It is clearly recommended that, within the limits of a real-life diet, saturated fatty acids and trans-UFA consumption should be as low as possible. This recommendation is especially true for the secondary prevention of coronary artery disease.[53] What a healthy diet in terms of balanced saturated fatty acids, mono-UFA, or poly-UFA intake really means for patients with HF remains unresolved.[54] Yet, because dietary fat intake seems to affect not only the development but also the progression of HF, clinicians routinely face the need to give advice on an adequate mixture of dietary fat.

Reduction of incidence of HF

A wealth of evidence is available to suggest that consumption of poly-UFAs in place of saturated fatty acids could reduce the rate of coronary artery disease,[55] resulting in a reduced incidence of HF. Hence, besides medical management of dyslipidemia in coronary artery disease, the implementation of a Mediterranean or DASH (Dietary Approaches to Stop Hypertension)-style diet,[56] rich in poly-UFA, is advised to reduce incidence of HF, and the American Heart Association supports an omega-6 poly-UFA intake of at least 5% to 10% of daily energy expenditure[57] in cardiovascular disease risk reduction in the general population.

Role of poly-UFA in HF

Aside from the prevention of HF, general recommendations for patients who need to lower their triglyceride level[58] include 2.0 to 4.0 g per day of docosahexaenoic acid and eicosapentaenoic acid. Substitution of fish-derived omega-3 poly-UFA in a dose of 4.0 g per day is known to decrease serum triglyceride concentrations by 25% to 30%, with accompanying increases of 5% to 10% in low-density lipoprotein cholesterol (LDL-C) and 1% to 3% in high-density lipoprotein cholesterol (HDL-C).[59] However, contrary to public belief, increased LDL-C levels are uncommon in HF, and some studies suggest that, similar to the obesity paradox, higher levels of LDL-C are associated with better survival in patients with HF.[60] This finding raises the questions of the role of poly-UFA in HF. The GISSI-HF (Gruppo Italiano per lo Studio della Sopravvivenza nellinfarto mIocardico - Heart Failure) investigators found a simple and safe treatment with omega-3 poly-UFA to provide a small beneficial advantage in terms of mortality and cardiovascular-related hospital admissions in patients with HF.[61] Although this finding was a milestone for nutritional advice in these patients, the large and coherent evidence on this matter has not been implemented in the clinical HF guidelines.

Role of mono-UFAs and long-chain-mono-UFAs in HF

In contrast to the array of evidence supporting the consumption of poly-UFA, mono-UFAs recently received less attention. Mono-UFAs, such as palmitoleic acid, are a central part of almost any diet and foods containing mono-UFAs are known to reduce LDL-C, although they may maintain or increase HDL-C. Together with poly-UFAs, mono-UFAs are generally considered a healthy type of fat. However, mono-UFAs are not to be confused with the important long-chained subgroup of fatty acids. Unlike mono-UFAs, which are predominantly oxidized in mitochondria, long-chain-mono-UFAs are oxidized in peroxisomes. Peroxisomal fatty acid oxidation of long-chain-mono-UFAs produces reactive oxygen species and has been associated with cardiotoxicity in animal models. A recent analysis by Imamura[62] of 2 representative, community-based, independent cohorts including 7271 patients found higher circulating levels of dietary 22:1 and 24:1 to be associated with incident HF. This finding, in combination with cellular studies and plausible biological pathways, including mitochondrial function and changes in energy metabolism, attributes a possible cardiotoxicity of long-chain-mono-UFAs in humans. A logical consequence would be to counsel patients seeking nutritional advice to drastically reduce consumption of long-chain-mono-UFAs. Fish oil supplements, olives, walnuts, flaxseed oil, sunflowers seeds, eggs, herring, or nuts are generally recommended as donors of beneficial fatty acids.[63] However, tablets are usual preferred by patients over lifestyle changes and that nutritional interventions should be introduced step by step into patients' lives.

Lipotoxicity and lipoprotection

In contrast to trends seen in the general population, obesity and hypercholesterolemia are associated with improved survival in HF. Patients with advanced or acutely decompensated HF often have low concentrations of LDL-C, which is associated with a poor prognosis in these patients.[64] This finding has not been fully understood, but sheds ambiguous light on interventional treatments aiming at a reduction of LDL-C and may bring the beneficial effects of cholesterol in HF[60] back onto the scientific agenda.

The important role of fatty acids in cardiac energetics, together with the reverse epidemiology of traditional cardiovascular risk factors in HF

reviewed by Kalantar-Zadeh,[46] may move our understanding away from lipotoxicity toward lipoprotection in the setting of HF.

Protein

Patients with HF require a greater amount of protein than healthy adults of the same age.[29] In addition, 20% to 30% of patients with HF suffer from hypoalbuminemia,[46] which was found to be independently associated with increased risk of death in patients with HF in a trial performed by Horwich and colleagues,[65] which investigated the effect of serum albumin level on survival in 1726 patients with advanced HF. Thus, provision of proteins may be considered a worthwhile target in HF care.

Direct supplementation of amino acids[23] may be considered more effective in patients with HF than the provision of protein and energy, because constituent amino acids are capable of being transformed into fat, protein, and carbohydrates and play a crucial role in metabolism. Although mere homocysteine, which is known to possess negative inotropic properties,[66] is usually not the first choice, branched-chain amino acids such as valine, leucine, and isoleucine[67] have been considered in the setting of cardiac cachexia.

L-Carnitine, the biologically active form of carnitine, a compound synthesized from the two amino acids lysine and methionine, plays an important role in cellular fatty acid and glucose metabolism. It is suggested to play a role in myocardial nutrient use[68] and observed to be decreased in HF.[69] Rizos[70] studied 80 patients with moderate to severe HF[71] caused by dilated cardiomyopathy, who were randomly assigned to receive either L-carnitine (2.0 g/d orally) or placebo. Survival analysis after nearly three years showed a significant ($P<.04$) survival benefit in the L-carnitine group. This encouraging interventional outcome, together with observational data, is suggestive of considerable potential for L-carnitine supplementation in patients with HF.

In contrast, rather than providing single substances, or specific substrates, promising results have also been achieved by provision of a multicompound and protein-rich high-caloric diet. Rozentryt and colleagues[72] reported significant clinical benefit in terms of body size, body composition, laboratory parameters, 6-minute walking distance, and quality of life by randomizing 29 patients to either a high-caloric (600 kcal), high-protein (20 g) oral nutritional supplement or placebo for a duration of 6 weeks and in addition to the patients' usual food. intake. These effects remained significant 12 weeks after the intervention was stopped.

Carbohydrates

As an important result of chronic overnutrition, especially high-sugar or high-fat feeding,[73] metabolic or diabetic cardiomyopathy is an emerging facet of HF. Of course, carbohydrates are an indispensable part of any diet and are recommended for building a nutritional foundation in the general population. Nevertheless, limited evidence exists concerning the role of carbohydrates as macronutrients in HF.

Impaired glucose tolerance or a diabetic metabolism are established risk factors for cardiovascular disease and have recently received increasing attention in the setting of HF. Hyperglycemia is known to promote atherosclerosis, associated with an altered cellular redox state, and results in increased oxidative stress.[74] Hence, aiming at euglycemia by tight glycemic control is considered a worthwhile treatment target and remains an important aspect in the care of patients with HF. However, for most clinicians, mild hyperglycemia is a tolerable state in hospitalized patients with HF, because the ubiquitous availability of glucose is desirable, especially in poorly perfused hypermetabolic tissues.

Further, insulin resistance, which is associated with reductions in cardiac insulin metabolic signaling, has recently been seen as an underestimated factor in the development of HF.[75] Endeavors to investigate the important interplay of relevant comorbidities and the heart[21] may eventually support dedicated evidence-based advice on carbohydrates in the setting of HF.

MICRONUTRIENTS

An impressive array of observational studies with various designs have investigated the dietary intake, adequacy, sufficiency, and status of micronutrients in the setting of HF. Vitamin D, thiamine, sodium, iron, ubiquinone, and selenium are among those that have received the most attention, but nearly all vitamins, electrolytes, and many chemical elements have been studied in this field.[35] Although focus was put on nutrient deficiency in the setting of HF in most cases, some attempts have been made to also understand increased serum levels of elements such as copper.[71]

The number of prospective, interventional studies or modest randomized, controlled trials evaluating the role of single micronutrients is limited. Adequately powered, randomized, controlled trials on relevant clinical outcomes such as mortality are not available in most cases. Nevertheless, some intellectually stimulating analyses, suggestive findings, and smart trials have delivered promising results and may pave the way for further investigations.

Vitamin D₃

In a case control study of 54 symptomatic patients with HF (NYHA functional class II–IV) and 34 healthy controls, significant reductions in circulating levels of both 25-hydroxyvitamin D (25[OH]D) ($P<.001$) and 1,25-dihydroxyvitamin D (calcitriol) ($P<.001$),[76] the biologically most relevant forms of vitamin D in humans, were reported in HF. This observation has been confirmed in several studies and led to the further investigation of association of vitamin D levels and prevalence of HF[77] in large population-based cohort-studies,[78] which has strongly supported the hypothesis that vitamin D might play a primary role in cardiovascular risk factors and disease. Other studies exist that could not reproduce or failed to show a relevant link between vitamin D and HF.[79] However, the Ludwigshafen Risk and Cardiovascular Health Study found low levels of 25(OH)D and calcitriol to be associated with prevalent myocardial dysfunction, deaths caused by HF (hazard ratio [HR] 2.84; 95% confidence interval [CI] 1.20–6.74), and sudden cardiac death (HR 5.05; 95% CI 2.13–11.97), indicating a strong prognostic relevance of vitamin D deficiency,[80] which has recently been confirmed by Gotsman[81] and colleagues, who not only found vitamin D deficiency to be an independent predictor of increased mortality in patients with HF (n = 3009) (HR 1.52; 95% CI 1.21–1.92; $P<.001$) but also vitamin D supplementation to be independently associated with reduced mortality in patients with HF (HR 0.68; 95% CI 0.54–0.85; $P<.0001$).

Highly relevant to patients' daily lives, vitamin D levels were also found to be associated with functional capacity. In a study of 101 with severe HF (NYHA functional class III or IV) higher levels of vitamin D were associated with better performance in cardiopulmonary stress tests (treadmill exercise, peak V_{O_2}) as an indicator of physical functioning capacity.[82] Fueled by the observational data on incidence, prognosis, and surrogate markers of morbidity, Witham and colleagues[83] conducted a randomized, parallel-group, double-blind, placebo-controlled trial in elderly patients with systolic HF with documented 25(OH)D levels less than 50 nmol/L. Although an increase in vitamin D levels could be observed, supplementation did not improve functional capacity or quality of life in these patients. However, natriuretic peptides did decrease in the interventional group. Prospective, interventional data on reduction of HF events or mortality for vitamin D supplementation are not available.

When advocating vitamin D, the unfavorable and potentially toxic side effects associated with its supplementation (ie, hypercalcemia) have to be kept in mind. The administration of chronic high-dose ($\geq$50,000 IU/d or higher) or single superdose ($\sim$865,000 IU) vitamin D supplements have been reported to be associated with complications, whereas chronic low-dose (400–4,000 IU/d) vitamin D is deemed tolerable. This finding shows not only the need for medical supervision but also for safety assessments in some situations and emphasizes the thin line between mere nutrient supplementation and active pharmaceutical treatment.

Thiamine

Thiamine is an essential B vitamin for many anabolic (ie, biosynthetic) and catabolic (ie, metabolic) processes. The association of HF, diuretic therapy, and thiamine deficiency was discussed earlier. The biologically most relevant form of thiamine is a product of thiamine and ATP, known as thiamine pyrophosphate. Thiamine pyrophosphate acts as a coenzyme in protein and carbohydrate metabolism and plays an important role in metabolic energetics.

Despite conflicting observational data on prevalence of thiamine deficiency in patients with HF and rationale of vitamin B_1 supplementation, a growing body of evidence supports its potential role in the interventional management of HF.

Shimon[84] found an improvement in left ventricular ejection fraction (LVEF) by 22% (0.27 $\pm$ 0.10 to 0.33 $\pm$ 0.11, P<.01) in a group of 30 hospitalized patients with HF randomized in a 1:1 fashion to a 1-week intravenous treatment with thiamine (200 mg/d) versus placebo, followed by a 6-week oral thiamine supplementation phase. Schoenenberger[85] evaluated the effect of a 28-day treatment with high-dose thiamine supplementation (300 mg/d) on LVEF in 9 patients with HF using a crossover design. Two patients (22%) were female, mean age was 56.7 $\pm$ 9.2 years in this study, baseline LVEF was 29.5% $\pm$ 2.4% in the thiamine and 29.5% $\pm$ 2.5% in the placebo group. Treatment resulted in a net increase of LVEF by 3.9% (P = .02). Although it remains unclear how this effect was mediated in detail, an improvement, albeit modest, of left ventricular systolic function by simple thiamine supplementation is an astonishing finding.

Further assessments of the role of B vitamins in the management of HF[86] are warranted, because vitamin B deficiency in hospitalized patients with HF is unrecognized.[87]

Sodium

Under continuous debate for decades, a strong link exists between sodium intake and blood pressure,[88] left ventricular hypertrophy,[89] cardiovascular disease,[90] other HF risk factors,[91] and even with incident HF per se.[92] Sodium is known to be highly involved in the maintenance of body fluid status, and excess sodium intake may therefore be linked to fluid overload and acute decompensation. Patients with HF are hence advised to restrict sodium intake to 2.0 g per day,[3] even although this is difficult in daily practice, considering that a deep-frozen pizza contains 2.0 to 8.0 g of sodium chloride. A simple guideline is usually to advise patients to not add extra salt when the dish is served on the table. Although some investigators conclude a higher sodium intake to be potentially harmful,[93] (1) the safest and most efficacious lower intake range and (2) whether that range would be applicable to all patients, or needs to be individualized, remains unknown.

Arcand and colleagues[94] prospectively enrolled 123 medically stable, ambulatory patients with systolic HF (mean $\pm$ SD age: 60 $\pm$ 13 years) and obtained estimates of dietary sodium and other nutrient intakes from 2 3-day food records. Median follow-up time was 3.0 years, mean ($\pm$ SD) sodium intakes were 1.4 $\pm$ 0.3, 2.4 $\pm$ 0.3, and 3.8 $\pm$ 0.8 g sodium per day in the lower, middle, and upper tertiles, respectively. These investigators found ambulatory patients with HF who consume higher amounts of sodium to be at greater risk of an acute decompensation HF event, hence putting stringent emphasis on sodium intake guidelines and showing the importance of dietary salt reduction.

Iron

The importance of iron deficiency has only recently received systematic research in HF, even although almost 80% of anemic patients with HF show some form of iron deficiency.[95] Even without anemia, iron deficiency is highly prevalent in patients with HF and its presence carries prognostic value.[96] In this context, iron deficiency is usually diagnosed using serum ferritin levels and transferrin saturation, but the cutoff values to correctly identify iron deficiency are different in patients with chronic disease such as HF and in healthy individuals.[97] Defining iron deficiency as either a serum ferritin level less than 100 µg/L (absolute iron deficiency) or ferritin level less than 300 µg/L in the presence of a transferrin saturation less than 20% (functional iron deficiency), the FAIR-HF (Ferinject Assessment in patients with IRon deficiency and chronic Heart Failure) investigators found treatment with intravenous ferric carboxymaltose in 459 patients with chronic HF and iron deficiency to be beneficial in terms of improved quality of life and 6-minute walking distance.[98] This effect was present regardless of the presence of anemia.[98] Intravenous iron supplementation may be preferable over oral supplementation, because chronic inflammatory processes and gut wall edema significantly hinder iron absorption in the duodenum.[99]

Ubiquinone, Coenzyme Q10

The main function of ubiquinone, also called coenzyme Q10 (CoQ10), is the biosynthesis of ATP through the mitochondrial electron transport chain. Highest CoQ10 concentrations have been found in the heart, and some studies even suggested a possible effect for CoQ10 in reduced hospitalization rates, dyspnea, and edema in patients with HF,[100,101] but these benefits have not been seen uniformly.[102,103] Because CoQ10 may improve LVEF in patients with HF,[104] Mortensen and colleagues (unpublished, 2011) are evaluating the supplementation of 2 mg/kg/d CoQ10 in 422 patients with HF over the course of the Q-SYMBIO (Coenzyme Q10 as adjunctive treatment of chronic heart failure: a randomised, double-blind, multicentre trial with focus on SYMptoms, BIOmarker status, and long-term outcome) outcomes trial.

Selenium

Observational evidence on selenium status in HF should not be considered coherent, but a spectrum of conclusive studies showed significant selenium deficiency in these patients.[35] Recommended daily intake of the essential trace element selenium is between 55 μg/d and 70 μg/d.[105] Yet, deLorgeril[53] revealed that dietary selenium intake is even lower in patients with HF than in healthy controls, leaving room for speculation on beneficial outcomes associated with interventional selenium. No trial on lone-standing, interventional selenium supplementation has investigated its potential in the setting of HF, but to determine the effect of micronutrients on exercise capacity and left ventricular function, de Lorgeril and colleagues[53] evaluated 21 consecutive patients with HF and 18 healthy age-matched and sex-matched controls regarding their dietary selenium intake and resulting blood levels. These investigators found peak Vo_2 (but not LVEF) to strongly correlate with blood selenium: $r = 0.76$ on univariable analysis (polynomial regression) and $r = 0.87$ ($P<.0005$) after adjustment for age, sex, and LVEF, and concluded that selenium may play a role in the clinical severity of the disease, rather than in the degree of left ventricular dysfunction. As selenium and selenoproteins are

crucial parts of the antioxidant systems of the human body, and functional capacity is an important aspect of any HF patient's daily life, selenium may be considered a promising treatment target. However, the setting of multiple rather than single-component supplementation remains to be evaluated.

Taking into account the report of decreased circulating levels of other micronutrients with antioxidant function such as zincum,[106,107] or the reported effect of vitamin E supplementation on the reduction of oxidative stress,[108] the potential of a balanced multiple-component, rather than single-component, micronutrient supplementation may be considered a promising endeavor.

SUMMARY

HF remains a disease with high morbidity and mortality accompanied by severe physical deterioration and clinically relevant nutritive imbalances. Several nutritional deficiencies have been documented in patients with HF and a group of supplements has been proposed and evaluated in these patients. Some prospective studies with nutritional supplementation have shown reasonable benefit in surrogate markers of morbidity (ie, NYHA functional class, quality of life, or improved LVEF). The best results have been achieved when documented nutrient deficiency has been treated. For the treatment of iron deficiency, regardless of the presence of manifest anemia, the intravenous supplementation of iron in the form of ferric carboxymaltose[98] has shown remarkable results, which have rapidly developed into routine clinical practice.[3] However, when nutritional deficiencies are not diagnosed or are underdiagnosed, evidence is less clear. Especially in the setting of acutely hospitalized patients, in whom increased oxidative stress and increasing consumption of antioxidants is discussed, and inflammation and reduction of stress are to be reduced, additional data are needed.

Although suggestive physiologic concepts exist for the biochemical effect of individual supplements, multicompound supplementation seems to be a tempting treatment option for the routine clinical setting, when detailed nutritional history taking and nutrient serum levels are not available. Witte and colleagues[109] investigated the effect of daily multicompound micronutrient supplementation consisting of vitamin D (10 μg), C (500 mg), and E (400 mg), thiamine (200 mg), selenium (50 μg), magnesium (150 mg), zinc (15 mg) CoQ10 (150 mg), and various other substances over the course of 9 months. This supplementation yielded a significant improvement ($P<.05$) in LVEF compared with placebo. Jeejeebhoy and colleagues[110] found a significant association of multiple-component nutritional supplementation with change in left ventricular end-diastolic volume (LVEDV) in patients with left ventricular dysfunction. LVEDV decreased by -7.5 ± 21.7 mL in the supplement group and increased by 10.0 ± 19.8 mL in the placebo group ($P = .037$).[110] How the reported effects are mediated remains unclear, but these clinical improvements in morbidity should not be neglected. Recently, Heyland and colleagues[111] reported to have randomly assigned 1223 critically ill adults (who had multiorgan failure, were receiving mechanical ventilation and prone to have odidative stress) to receive a supplementation of glutamine, antioxidants, both, or placebo. At 28 days, there was a trend towards increased mortality among patients who received glutamine (0.35 g/kg/day intravenously and 30 g/d enterally), as compared with patients who did not receive glutamine but matching placebo solutions (32.4% vs 27.2%; adjusted odds ratio, 1.28; 95% CI, 1.00 to 1.64; $P = .05$). In-hospital mortality and mortality at 6 months were significantly higher among patients who received glutamine than among patients who did not.

In addition, patients were randomly assigned to daily receive antioxidants (500 μg of selenium intravenously plus selenium (300 μg), zincum (20 mg), beta carotene (10 mg), vitamine E (500 mg), and vitamin C (1500 mg) enterally) or matching placebo. While supplementation of glutamine was found harmful, antioxidant supplementation was not associated with any effect on study outcomes.[111] Although this trial does not focus on the specific setting of HF, Heyland's findings may either reflect the true lack of prognostic usefulness of antioxidants in the critically ill; or alternatively may be seen due to compounding, dose, and method of administration in these patients.[111]

To our knowledge, no single conclusive clinical trial on dedicated nutritional supplementation has reported improved outcomes or survival in patients with HF. Only limited data on safety, pharmaceutical interactions, and adverse effects of nutrient supplementation are available. In this light, improvements in LVEF and NYHA functional class after a short-term follow-up may seem promising at first hand, but having learned a tough lesson from clinical trials on positive inotropic agents, the evaluation of long-term effects including morbidity and mortality remains crucial for patient management.

Therefore, aside from a pragmatic clinical approach to replenishment of documented deficiencies in the setting of acute or hospitalized HF,[74] nutritional supplements are not recommended for the treatment of HF.[4] Further investigations that assess safety and efficacy and close the gap in evidence regarding patients with HF are needed.

ACKNOWLEDGMENT

Preparation of this manuscript has partly been supported by the European Union's Seventh Framework Programme [FP7/2007–2013] under grant agreement n° 241558 (SICA-HF).

REFERENCES

1. Writing Group Members, Lloyd-Jones D, Adams RJ, Brown TM, et al. Heart disease and stroke statistics–2010 update: a report from the American Heart Association. Circulation 2010; 121(7):e46–215.
2. Cowie MR, Mosterd A, Wood DA, et al. The epidemiology of heart failure. Eur Heart J 1997;18(2): 208–25.
3. McMurray JJ, Adamopoulos S, Anker SD, et al. ESC guidelines for the diagnosis and treatment of acute and chronic heart failure 2012: The Task Force for the Diagnosis and Treatment of Acute and Chronic Heart Failure 2012 of the European Society of Cardiology. Developed in collaboration with the Heart Failure Association (HFA) of the ESC. Eur J Heart Fail 2012;14(8):803–69.
4. Hunt SA, Abraham WT, Chin MH, et al. 2009 focused update incorporated into the ACC/AHA 2005 guidelines for the diagnosis and management of heart failure in adults: a report of the American College of Cardiology Foundation/American Heart Association Task Force on Practice Guidelines: developed in collaboration with the International Society for Heart and Lung Transplantation. Circulation 2009;119(14):e391–479.
5. Stewart S, MacIntyre K, Hole DJ, et al. More 'malignant' than cancer? Five-year survival following a first admission for heart failure. Eur J Heart Fail 2001;3(3):315–22.
6. Anker SD, Ponikowski P, Varney S, et al. Wasting as independent risk factor for mortality in chronic heart failure. Lancet 1997;349(9058):1050–3.
7. Kalantar-Zadeh K, Block G, Horwich T, et al. Reverse epidemiology of conventional cardiovascular risk factors in patients with chronic heart failure. J Am Coll Cardiol 2004;43(8):1439–44.
8. Trippel TD, Lenk J, Stahn A, et al. Multi compartment body composition analysis in chronic heart failure. Eur Heart J 2012;33(Abstract Supplement):883.
9. Sarma S, Gheorghiade M. Nutritional assessment and support of the patient with acute heart failure. Curr Opin Crit Care 2010;16(5):413–8.

10. von Haehling S, Lainscak M, Springer J, et al. Cardiac cachexia: a systematic overview. Pharmacol Ther 2009;121(3):227–52.

11. Filippatos GS, Anker SD, Kremastinos DT. Pathophysiology of peripheral muscle wasting in cardiac cachexia. Curr Opin Clin Nutr Metab Care 2005; 8(3):249–54.

12. Anker MS, von Haehling S, Springer J, et al. Highlights of the mechanistic and therapeutic cachexia and sarcopenia research 2010 to 2012 and their relevance for cardiology. Int J Cardiol 2013; 162(2):73–6.

13. Davos CH, Doehner W, Rauchhaus M, et al. Body mass and survival in patients with chronic heart failure without cachexia: the importance of obesity. J Card Fail 2003;9(1):29–35.

14. Gastelurrutia P, Lupon J, Domingo M, et al. Usefulness of body mass index to characterize nutritional status in patients with heart failure. Am J Cardiol 2011;108(8):1166–70.

15. Strassburg S, Springer J, Anker SD. Muscle wasting in cardiac cachexia. Int J Biochem Cell Biol 2005;37(10):1938–47.

16. Sakuma K, Yamaguchi A. Sarcopenia and cachexia: the adaptations of negative regulators of skeletal muscle mass. J Cachexia Sarcopenia Muscle 2012;3(2):77–94.

17. von Haehling S. The muscle in dire straits: mechanisms of wasting in heart failure. Circulation 2012; 125(22):2686–8.

18. Fearon K, Evans WJ, Anker SD. Myopenia–a new universal term for muscle wasting. J Cachexia Sarcopenia Muscle 2011;2(1):1–3.

19. Morley JE, Abbatecola AM, Argiles JM, et al. Sarcopenia with limited mobility: an international consensus. J Am Med Dir Assoc 2011;12(6): 403–9.

20. Fülster S, Tacke M, Sandek A, et al. Muscle wasting in patients with chronic heart failure: results from the studies investigating co-morbidities aggravating heart failure (SICA-HF). Eur Heart J 2013; 34(7):512–9.

21. von Haehling S, Lainscak M, Doehner W, et al. Diabetes mellitus, cachexia and obesity in heart failure: rationale and design of the Studies Investigating Co-morbidities Aggravating Heart Failure (SICA-HF). J Cachexia Sarcopenia Muscle 2010;1(2): 187–94.

22. Aquilani R, Opasich C, Gualco A, et al. Adequate energy-protein intake is not enough to improve nutritional and metabolic status in muscle-depleted patients with chronic heart failure. Eur J Heart Fail 2008;10(11):1127–35.

23. Aquilani R, Viglio S, Iadarola P, et al. Oral amino acid supplements improve exercise capacities in elderly patients with chronic heart failure. Am J Cardiol 2008;101(11A):104E–10E.

24. Macchi A, Franzoni I, Buzzetti F. The role of essential amino acid supplementation in chronic heart failure [abstract]. Eur Heart J 2009; 30(Suppl):869.

25. Carr JG, Stevenson LW, Walden JA, et al. Prevalence and hemodynamic correlates of malnutrition in severe congestive heart failure secondary to ischemic or idiopathic dilated cardiomyopathy. Am J Cardiol 1989;63(11):709–13.

26. Freeman LM, Roubenoff R. The nutrition implications of cardiac cachexia. Nutr Rev 1994;52(10): 340–7.

27. Grossniklaus DA, O'Brien MC, Clark PC, et al. Nutrient intake in heart failure patients. J Cardiovasc Nurs 2008;23(4):357–63.

28. Gibbs CR, Jackson G, Lip GY. ABC of heart failure. Non-drug management. BMJ 2000;320(7231): 366–9.

29. Lennie TA, Moser DK, Heo S, et al. Factors influencing food intake in patients with heart failure: a comparison with healthy elders. J Cardiovasc Nurs 2006;21(2):123–9.

30. Sandek A, Bauditz J, Swidsinski A, et al. Altered intestinal function in patients with chronic heart failure. J Am Coll Cardiol 2007;50(16):1561–9.

31. King D, Smith ML, Chapman TJ, et al. Fat malabsorption in elderly patients with cardiac cachexia. Age Ageing 1996;25(2):144–9.

32. King D, Smith ML, Lye M. Gastro-intestinal protein loss in elderly patients with cardiac cachexia. Age Ageing 1996;25(3):221–3.

33. Arutyunov GP, Kostyukevich OI, Serov RA, et al. Collagen accumulation and dysfunctional mucosal barrier of the small intestine in patients with chronic heart failure. Int J Cardiol 2008;125(2):240–5.

34. Sandek A, Bjarnason I, Volk HD, et al. Studies on bacterial endotoxin and intestinal absorption function in patients with chronic heart failure. Int J Cardiol 2012;157(1):80–5.

35. McKeag NA, McKinley MC, Woodside JV, et al. The role of micronutrients in heart failure. J Acad Nutr Diet 2012;112(6):870–86.

36. Dunn SP, Bleske B, Dorsch M, et al. Nutrition and heart failure: impact of drug therapies and management strategies. Nutr Clin Pract 2009;24(1):60–75.

37. Nieminen MS, Brutsaert D, Dickstein K, et al. EuroHeart Failure Survey II (EHFS II): a survey on hospitalized acute heart failure patients: description of population. Eur Heart J 2006;27(22):2725–36.

38. Yue QY, Beermann B, Lindstrom B, et al. No difference in blood thiamine diphosphate levels between Swedish Caucasian patients with congestive heart failure treated with furosemide and patients without heart failure. J Intern Med 1997;242(6):491–5.

39. Hardig L, Daae C, Dellborg M, et al. Reduced thiamine phosphate, but not thiamine diphosphate, in erythrocytes in elderly patients with congestive

heart failure treated with furosemide. J Intern Med 2000;247(5):597–600.

40. Suter PM, Haller J, Hany A, et al. Diuretic use: a risk for subclinical thiamine deficiency in elderly patients. J Nutr Health Aging 2000;4(2):69–71.

41. Sica DA. Loop diuretic therapy, thiamine balance, and heart failure. Congest Heart Fail 2007;13(4): 244–7.

42. Rosenberg J, Gustafsson F, Galatius S, et al. Combination therapy with metolazone and loop diuretics in outpatients with refractory heart failure: an observational study and review of the literature. Cardiovasc Drugs Ther 2005;19(4): 301–6.

43. Poehlman ET, Scheffers J, Gottlieb SS, et al. Increased resting metabolic rate in patients with congestive heart failure. Ann Intern Med 1994; 121(11):860–2.

44. Toth MJ, Matthews DE. Whole-body protein metabolism in chronic heart failure: relationship to anabolic and catabolic hormones. JPEN J Parenter Enteral Nutr 2006;30(3):194–201.

45. Witte KK, Clark AL. Micronutrients and their supplementation in chronic cardiac failure. An update beyond theoretical perspectives. Heart Fail Rev 2006;11(1):65–74.

46. Kalantar-Zadeh K, Anker SD, Horwich TB, et al. Nutritional and anti-inflammatory interventions in chronic heart failure. Am J Cardiol 2008;101(11A): 89E–103E.

47. Bourdel-Marchasson I, Emeriau JP. Nutritional strategy in the management of heart failure in adults. Am J Cardiovasc Drugs 2001;1(5): 363–73.

48. Turer AT. Using metabolomics to assess myocardial metabolism and energetics in heart failure. J Mol Cell Cardiol 2013;55:12–8.

49. Nagoshi T, Yoshimura M, Rosano GM, et al. Optimization of cardiac metabolism in heart failure. Curr Pharm Des 2011;17(35):3846–53.

50. Ardehali H, Sabbah HN, Burke MA, et al. Targeting myocardial substrate metabolism in heart failure: potential for new therapies. Eur J Heart Fail 2012; 14(2):120–9.

51. Shah SH, Kraus WE, Newgard CB. Metabolomic profiling for the identification of novel biomarkers and mechanisms related to common cardiovascular diseases: form and function. Circulation 2012; 126(9):1110–20.

52. Lopaschuk GD, Ussher JR, Folmes CD, et al. Myocardial fatty acid metabolism in health and disease. Physiol Rev 2010;90(1):207–58.

53. de Lorgeril M, Salen P, Accominotti M, et al. Dietary and blood antioxidants in patients with chronic heart failure. Insights into the potential importance of selenium in heart failure. Eur J Heart Fail 2001; 3(6):661–9.

54. Stanley WC, Dabkowski ER, Ribeiro RF Jr, et al. Dietary fat and heart failure: moving from lipotoxicity to lipoprotection. Circ Res 2012;110(5):764–76.

55. Mozaffarian D, Micha R, Wallace S. Effects on coronary heart disease of increasing polyunsaturated fat in place of saturated fat: a systematic review and meta-analysis of randomized controlled trials. PLoS Med 2010;7(3):e1000252.

56. Levitan EB, Wolk A, Mittleman MA. Consistency with the DASH diet and incidence of heart failure. Arch Intern Med 2009;169(9):851–7.

57. Harris WS, Mozaffarian D, Rimm E, et al. Omega-6 fatty acids and risk for cardiovascular disease: a science advisory from the American Heart Association Nutrition Subcommittee of the Council on Nutrition, Physical Activity, and Metabolism; Council on Cardiovascular Nursing; and Council on Epidemiology and Prevention. Circulation 2009;119(6): 902–7.

58. Kris-Etherton PM, Harris WS, Appel LJ, et al. Fish consumption, fish oil, omega-3 fatty acids, and cardiovascular disease. Circulation 2002;106(21): 2747–57.

59. Harris WS. n-3 fatty acids and serum lipoproteins: human studies. Am J Clin Nutr 1997;65(Suppl 5): 1645S–54S.

60. Rauchhaus M, Clark AL, Doehner W, et al. The relationship between cholesterol and survival in patients with chronic heart failure. J Am Coll Cardiol 2003;42(11):1933–40.

61. Gissi-HF Investigators, Tavazzi L, Maggioni AP, Marchioli R, et al. Effect of n-3 polyunsaturated fatty acids in patients with chronic heart failure (the GISSI-HF trial): a randomised, double-blind, placebo-controlled trial. Lancet 2008;372(9645): 1223–30.

62. Imamura F, Lemaitre RN, King IB, et al. Long-chain monounsaturated fatty acids and incidence of congestive heart failure in 2 prospective cohorts. Circulation 2013;127(14):1512–21.

63. Azhar G, Wei JY. Nutrition and cardiac cachexia. Curr Opin Clin Nutr Metab Care 2006;9(1):18–23.

64. Kahn MR, Kosmas CE, Wagman G, et al. Low-density lipoprotein levels in patients with acute heart failure. Congest Heart Fail 2013;19(2):85–91.

65. Horwich TB, Kalantar-Zadeh K, MacLellan RW, et al. Albumin levels predict survival in patients with systolic heart failure. Am Heart J 2008; 155(5):883–9.

66. Kennedy RH, Owings R, Shekhawat N, et al. Acute negative inotropic effects of homocysteine are mediated via the endothelium. Am J Physiol Heart Circ Physiol 2004;287(2):H812–7.

67. Laviano A, Muscaritoli M, Cascino A, et al. Branched-chain amino acids: the best compromise to achieve anabolism? Curr Opin Clin Nutr Metab Care 2005;8(4):408–14.

68. Calvani M, Reda E, Arrigoni-Martelli E. Regulation by carnitine of myocardial fatty acid and carbohydrate metabolism under normal and pathological conditions. Basic Res Cardiol 2000;95(2):75–83.

69. Regitz V, Shug AL, Fleck E. Defective myocardial carnitine metabolism in congestive heart failure secondary to dilated cardiomyopathy and to coronary, hypertensive and valvular heart diseases. Am J Cardiol 1990;65(11):755–60.

70. Rizos I. Three-year survival of patients with heart failure caused by dilated cardiomyopathy and L-carnitine administration. Am Heart J 2000; 139(2 Pt 3):S120–3.

71. Malek F, Dvorak J, Jiresova E, et al. Difference of baseline serum copper levels between groups of patients with different one year mortality and morbidity and chronic heart failure. Cent Eur J Public Health 2003;11(4):198–201.

72. Rozentryt P, von Haehling S, Lainscak M, et al. The effects of a high-caloric protein-rich oral nutritional supplement in patients with chronic heart failure and cachexia on quality of life, body composition, and inflammation markers: a randomized, double-blind pilot study. J Cachexia Sarcopenia Muscle 2010;1(1):35–42.

73. Mandavia CH, Pulakat L, DeMarco V, et al. Overnutrition and metabolic cardiomyopathy. Metabolism 2012;61(9):1205–10.

74. Meltzer JS, Moitra VK. The nutritional and metabolic support of heart failure in the intensive care unit. Curr Opin Clin Nutr Metab Care 2008;11(2): 140–6.

75. Aroor AR, Mandavia CH, Sowers JR. Insulin resistance and heart failure: molecular mechanisms. Heart Fail Clin 2012;8(4):609–17.

76. Zittermann A, Schleithoff SS, Tenderich G, et al. Low vitamin D status: a contributing factor in the pathogenesis of congestive heart failure? J Am Coll Cardiol 2003;41(1):105–12.

77. Kim DH, Sabour S, Sagar UN, et al. Prevalence of hypovitaminosis D in cardiovascular diseases (from the National Health and Nutrition Examination Survey 2001 to 2004). Am J Cardiol 2008;102(11): 1540–4.

78. Anderson JL, May HT, Horne BD, et al. Relation of vitamin D deficiency to cardiovascular risk factors, disease status, and incident events in a general healthcare population. Am J Cardiol 2010;106(7): 963–8.

79. Bolland MJ, Bacon CJ, Horne AM, et al. Vitamin D insufficiency and health outcomes over 5 y in older women. Am J Clin Nutr 2010;91(1):82–9.

80. Pilz S, Marz W, Wellnitz B, et al. Association of vitamin D deficiency with heart failure and sudden cardiac death in a large cross-sectional study of patients referred for coronary angiography. J Clin Endocrinol Metab 2008;93(10):3927–35.

81. Gotsman I, Shauer A, Zwas DR, et al. Vitamin D deficiency is a predictor of reduced survival in patients with heart failure; vitamin D supplementation improves outcome. Eur J Heart Fail 2012;14(4): 357–66.

82. Shane E, Mancini D, Aaronson K, et al. Bone mass, vitamin D deficiency, and hyperparathyroidism in congestive heart failure. Am J Med 1997;103(3): 197–207.

83. Witham MD, Crighton LJ, Gillespie ND, et al. The effects of vitamin D supplementation on physical function and quality of life in older patients with heart failure: a randomized controlled trial. Circ Heart Fail 2010;3(2):195–201.

84. Shimon I, Almog S, Vered Z, et al. Improved left ventricular function after thiamine supplementation in patients with congestive heart failure receiving long-term furosemide therapy. Am J Med 1995; 98(5):485–90.

85. Schoenenberger AW, Schoenenberger-Berzins R, der Maur CA, et al. Thiamine supplementation in symptomatic chronic heart failure: a randomized, double-blind, placebo-controlled, cross-over pilot study. Clin Res Cardiol 2012;101(3):159–64.

86. Azizi-Namini P, Ahmed M, Yan AT, et al. The role of B vitamins in the management of heart failure. Nutr Clin Pract 2012;27(3):363–74.

87. Keith ME, Walsh NA, Darling PB, et al. B-vitamin deficiency in hospitalized patients with heart failure. J Am Diet Assoc 2009;109(8):1406–10.

88. He FJ, MacGregor GA. Effect of longer-term modest salt reduction on blood pressure. Cochrane Database Syst Rev 2004;(3):CD004937.

89. Jula AM, Karanko HM. Effects on left ventricular hypertrophy of long-term nonpharmacological treatment with sodium restriction in mild-to-moderate essential hypertension. Circulation 1994;89(3): 1023–31.

90. Cook NR, Cutler JA, Obarzanek E, et al. Long term effects of dietary sodium reduction on cardiovascular disease outcomes: observational follow-up of the trials of hypertension prevention (TOHP). BMJ 2007;334(7599):885–8.

91. Strazzullo P, D'Elia L, Kandala NB, et al. Salt intake, stroke, and cardiovascular disease: meta-analysis of prospective studies. BMJ 2009;339:b4567.

92. He J, Ogden LG, Bazzano LA, et al. Dietary sodium intake and incidence of congestive heart failure in overweight US men and women: first National Health and Nutrition Examination Survey Epidemiologic Follow-up Study. Arch Intern Med 2002; 162(14):1619–24.

93. Gupta D, Georgiopoulou VV, Kalogeropoulos AP, et al. Dietary sodium intake in heart failure. Circulation 2012;126(4):479–85.

94. Arcand J, Ivanov J, Sasson A, et al. A high-sodium diet is associated with acute decompensated heart

failure in ambulatory heart failure patients: a prospective follow-up study. Am J Clin Nutr 2011; 93(2):332–7.

95. Ezekowitz JA, McAlister FA, Armstrong PW. Anemia is common in heart failure and is associated with poor outcomes: insights from a cohort of 12 065 patients with new-onset heart failure. Circulation 2003;107(2):223–5.

96. Jankowska EA, Rozentryt P, Witkowska A, et al. Iron deficiency predicts impaired exercise capacity in patients with systolic chronic heart failure. J Card Fail 2011;17(11):899–906.

97. von Haehling S, Jankowska EA, Ponikowski P, et al. Anemia in heart failure: an overview of current concepts. Future Cardiol 2011;7(1):119–29.

98. Anker SD, Comin Colet J, Filippatos G, et al. Ferric carboxymaltose in patients with heart failure and iron deficiency. N Engl J Med 2009;361(25):2436–48.

99. von Haehling S, Anker MS, Jankowska EA, et al. Anemia in chronic heart failure: can we treat? What to treat? Heart Fail Rev 2012;17(2):203–10.

100. Baggio E, Gandini R, Plancher AC, et al. Italian multicenter study on the safety and efficacy of coenzyme Q10 as adjunctive therapy in heart failure. CoQ10 Drug Surveillance Investigators. Mol Aspects Med 1994;15(Suppl):s287–94.

101. Hofman-Bang C, Rehnqvist N, Swedberg K, et al. Coenzyme Q10 as an adjunctive in the treatment of chronic congestive heart failure. The Q10 Study Group. J Card Fail 1995;1(2):101–7.

102. Watson PS, Scalia GM, Galbraith A, et al. Lack of effect of coenzyme Q on left ventricular function in patients with congestive heart failure. J Am Coll Cardiol 1999;33(6):1549–52.

103. Miller KL, Liebowitz RS, Newby LK. Complementary and alternative medicine in cardiovascular disease: a review of biologically based approaches. Am Heart J 2004;147(3):401–11.

104. Fotino AD, Thompson-Paul AM, Bazzano LA. Effect of coenzyme Q(1)(0) supplementation on heart failure: a meta-analysis. Am J Clin Nutr 2013;97(2):268–75.

105. Fairweather-Tait SJ, Bao Y, Broadley MR, et al. Selenium in human health and disease. Antioxid Redox Signal 2011;14(7):1337–83.

106. Salehifar E, Shokrzadeh M, Ghaemian A, et al. The study of Cu and Zn serum levels in idiopathic dilated cardiomyopathy (IDCMP) patients and its comparison with healthy volunteers. Biol Trace Elem Res 2008;125(2):97–108.

107. Shokrzadeh M, Ghaemian A, Salehifar E, et al. Serum zinc and copper levels in ischemic cardiomyopathy. Biol Trace Elem Res 2009;127(2):116–23.

108. Ghatak A, Brar MJ, Agarwal A, et al. Oxy free radical system in heart failure and therapeutic role of oral vitamin E. Int J Cardiol 1996;57(2):119–27.

109. Witte KK, Nikitin NP, Parker AC, et al. The effect of micronutrient supplementation on quality-of-life and left ventricular function in elderly patients with chronic heart failure. Eur Heart J 2005;26(21):2238–44.

110. Jeejeebhoy F, Keith M, Freeman M, et al. Nutritional supplementation with MyoVive repletes essential cardiac myocyte nutrients and reduces left ventricular size in patients with left ventricular dysfunction. Am Heart J 2002;143(6):1092–100.

111. Heyland D, Muscedere J, Wischmeyer PE, et al. A randomized trial of glutamine and antioxidants in critically ill patients. N Engl J Med 2013;368:1489–97.

Noncardiac Comorbidities and Acute Heart Failure Patients

Robert J. Mentz, MD*, G. Michael Felker, MD, MHS

KEYWORDS

- Heart failure • Comorbidities • COPD • Renal disease • Diabetes • Anemia
- Sleep-disordered breathing

KEY POINTS

- The acute heart failure (AHF) population represents a heterogeneous cohort with multiple interrelated noncardiovascular comorbidities.
- Chronic obstructive pulmonary disease, renal disease, diabetes, sleep apnea, and anemia impact the clinical characteristics and outcomes of patients with AHF and complicate in-hospital management.
- Attention to the diagnosis and management of comorbidities in patients with AHF may improve patient outcomes.

INTRODUCTION

Patients with heart failure (HF) commonly have multiple comorbid diseases that complicate management. Risk factors, such as smoking, obesity, and advanced age, increase the burden of noncardiovascular comorbidities including chronic obstructive pulmonary disease (COPD), sleep apnea, and diabetes mellitus (DM). Registry and trial data suggest that these comorbidities are present in more than 30% of patients with HF (Table 1).[1–3] In addition, patients with HF frequently have kidney disease and evidence of liver dysfunction, which may worsen at the time of HF hospitalization and adversely impact inpatient management and clinical course.[4,5] In one study of Medicare patients, nearly 40% of elderly patients with HF had five or more noncardiac comorbidities and this group accounted for most total hospital days.[6] Thus, the acute HF (AHF) population represents a heterogeneous cohort with multiple interrelated noncardiovascular comorbidities (Fig. 1).

Despite recent advances in the care of patients with chronic HF, the AHF population remains at high risk for adverse events postdischarge. The presence of comorbidities in patients with AHF has been associated with significantly increased morbidity and mortality.[2,7] The risk of hospitalization markedly increases with the number of noncardiac chronic conditions.[6] Rehospitalization rates after AHF are nearly as high for noncardiovascular causes as for HF.[8] Once hospitalized, comorbid pulmonary, renal, and liver dysfunction along with sleep apnea syndromes complicate the management of dyspnea and congestion in AHF (Fig. 2). This article summarizes the impact of comorbidities on the characteristics, treatment, and outcomes of patients with AHF. Attention to the diagnosis and management of these conditions in patients with AHF may help to improve patient outcomes.

Funding Support: None.

Disclosures: None.

Division of Cardiology, Department of Medicine, Duke University Medical Center, 2301 Erwin Road, Durham, NC 27710, USA

* Corresponding author. Duke University Medical Center, 2301 Erwin Road, Durham, NC 27710.

E-mail address: robert.mentz@duke.edu

1551-7136/13/$ – see front matter © 2013 Elsevier Inc. All rights reserved.

Table 1
Prevalence of noncardiovascular comorbidities in patients with acute heart failure

	ADHERE (n = 187,565)	OPTIMIZE-HF (n = 48,612)	EHFS II (n = 3580)
Region	United States	United States	Europe
Age (y)	75	73	70
Male (%)	48	48	61
Preserved ejection fraction (%)	53	51	52
Medical history			
COPD	31	28	19
Chronic renal insufficiency	30	20	17
Diabetes mellitus	44	42	33
Anemia	53	18	15
Depression	—	11	—
Liver disease	—	2	—

Abbreviations: ADHERE, Acute Decompensated Heart Failure National Registry; COPD, chronic obstructive pulmonary disease; EHFS II, EuroHeart Failure Survey II; OPTIMIZE-HF, Organized Program to Initiate Lifesaving Treatment in Hospitalized Patients with Heart Failure.

COPD

COPD is present in approximately 30% of patients with HF.[9] Patients with HF with COPD tend to have an increased burden of other comorbidities, including hypertension, atrial fibrillation, and coronary artery disease (CAD), compared with those without COPD.[10] The underlying pathophysiology may be caused by the shared risk factor of smoking with low-grade systemic inflammation accelerating disease progression.[11] Patients with AHF with COPD tend to have lower blood pressure,

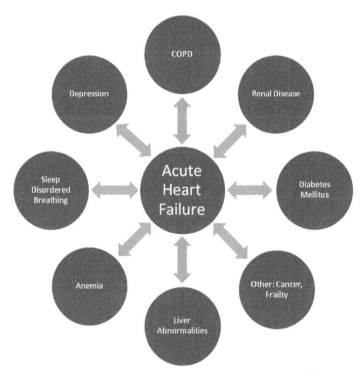

Fig. 1. Interrelated noncardiovascular comorbidities in patients with acute heart failure. COPD, chronic obstructive pulmonary disease.

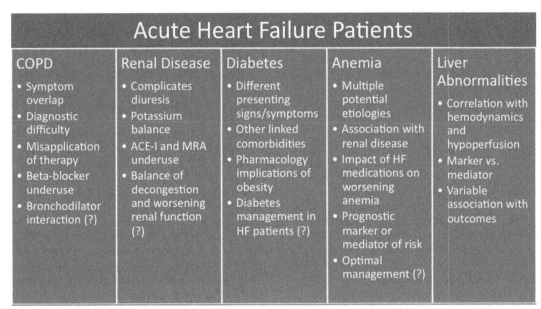

Fig. 2. Key characteristics associated with different noncardiovascular comorbidities in patients with acute heart failure. ACE-I, angiotensin-converting enzyme inhibitor; COPD, chronic obstructive pulmonary disease; MRA, mineralocorticoid receptor antagonist.

higher creatinine, and underuse of angiotensin-converting enzyme (ACE) inhibitors and mineralocorticoid receptor antagonists (MRAs).[12,13] They are less likely to receive β-blockers compared with those without COPD[10] because of concerns about precipitating bronchospasm.[14–16] The primary effect of COPD may be increased noncardiovascular mortality in the AHF setting[12] with similar outcomes after hospital discharge.[13] However, other studies have suggested an increased long-term risk for morbidity[10] and mortality[6] associated with COPD in chronic HF.

The overlapping symptom of dyspnea with both diseases may confound appropriate diagnosis at the time of disease exacerbation and may lead to misapplication of therapy. Given the discordant β receptor effects of the different disease treatments, a patient's symptoms and outcome could be adversely affected by the treatment of the comorbid disease. For instance, there are observational data demonstrating potential cardiovascular risks with β_2 agonists in patients with HF.[16] However, because worse outcomes in previous studies may be attributed to confounding by indication or COPD severity rather than an adverse effect of therapy, these results should be viewed as exploratory. Alternatively, worsening of one disease process may adversely impact the other disease such that concomitant exacerbations may contribute to clinical deterioration during hospitalization. Careful evaluation of evidence for congestion, edema, and bronchospasm along

with natriuretic peptide levels may help determine the relative contribution of each disease process. Thus, therapy can be appropriately targeted in an individual patient to improve his or her symptoms and clinical course.

Anticholinergic bronchodilators may have a more reassuring safety profile compared with β-agonists and may be the preferred first-line agents for patients with COPD with comorbid HF.[14] Conversely, β-blockers do not worsen airway function in most patients with COPD in the chronic setting,[17] yet less is known about their use during hospitalization for pulmonary exacerbation. As a patient's pulmonary exacerbation resolves and there is no evidence of ongoing bronchospasm, it may be possible to initiate β-blockers in patients with HF with COPD. The hospitalized setting may provide the optimal environment for initiation of these therapies, because the patient can be closely monitored for adverse events. Dosages should be carefully titrated to the doses used in clinical trials or to the maximally tolerated dose with monitoring commensurate to the patient's presentation and clinical course. The decision to use a cardioselective versus noncardioselective β-blocker in these patients may not impact outcomes.[10,18]

Taken together, these data highlight the complexities of treating patients with concomitant HF and COPD, and suggest increased risk when the diseases are present together. Because trials investigating the management of patients with COPD have generally excluded patients with significant HF, and vice versa, limited data exist on the management of these patients. We have recently proposed a randomized trial designed to enroll patients with significant COPD and HF to determine the risks and benefits of different bronchodilator and β-blocker strategies.[16]

RENAL DISEASE

Chronic kidney disease (CKD) is present in approximately 30% of patients with HF. The interdependence of the heart and the kidney is captured in the cardiorenal syndrome.[4,19] Risk factors for the development of HF and vascular disease (eg, hypertension and diabetes) contribute to the prevalence of renal disease in these patients. Patients with AHF with renal dysfunction tend to be older, with lower blood pressure, higher brain natriuretic peptide levels, and more clinical signs of HF.[20] Renal dysfunction is an established risk factor for adverse events in patients with HF.[21,22] The ADHERE registry revealed that greater than half of patients with AHF had at least moderate renal insufficiency (estimated glomerular filtration rate [eGFR] <60 mL/min/1.73 m^2) on admission, which was associated with increased mortality.[23]

CKD impacts baseline medication use in patients with HF and complicates in-hospital management. ACE inhibitors and MRAs are frequently underused in patients with HF with renal disease because of concerns about worsening GFR and hyperkalemia.[20] Of the limited data available on the use of ACE inhibitors in patients with AHF who experience worsening renal failure (WRF), an association between their use and WRF has not been demonstrated.[24,25] Recommendations are to use ACE inhibitors and MRAs with caution in those with reduced eGFR and to avoid these classes when eGFR falls below 30 mL/min/1.73 m^2 or in patients with hyperkalemia.[26] In the setting of dynamic fluctuations in renal function during AHF, the degree of monitoring and discontinuation of these agents should be determined based on the clinical situation.[27] Similar to the initiation of β-blockers in patients with COPD with HF, the in-hospital setting may be an ideal time to start ACE inhibitors and MRAs in patients with renal dysfunction after clinical stabilization.

CKD may complicate the ability to successfully decongest patients with AHF and increases the likelihood of experiencing WRF.[28] Renal disease may necessitate increased diuretic dosing to achieve an effect in AHF such that an initial management step is to challenge the patient with higher doses of loop diuretics. Adequate decongestion in this patient population may also be limited by underlying diuretic resistance and the addition of a thiazide diuretic may augment diuresis. Notably, baseline renal dysfunction is a predictor of WRF during AHF, which has been associated with increased mortality.[29–32]

However, recent data exploring the implications of WRF in patients with AHF have questioned the association with worse outcomes. For instance, transient WRF during AHF hospitalization may not impact postdischarge outcomes[33,34] and aggressive fluid removal involving hemoconcentration may be associated with lower mortality despite WRF.[34] Data from the DOSE study suggested that higher doses of diuretics are more efficacious in relieving congestion, at the cost of WRF that does not seem to have long-term consequences.[35] Given that persistent congestion is a predictor of adverse outcomes,[36] transient WRF may be acceptable in exchange for decongestion. Thus, baseline CKD is associated with worse outcomes in patients with AHF, but management strategies that optimize decongestion and prioritize the initiation of guideline-recommended HF medications may lead to improved outcomes.

DIABETES

Approximately 40% of patients with AHF have DM.[1] Patients with AHF with DM are more likely to have hypertension, obesity, ischemic etiology, kidney disease, anemia, and vascular disease.[37–39] In an observational AHF study, patients with DM tended to more frequently present with acute pulmonary edema or acute coronary syndrome compared with those without DM.[38] Although DM is associated with increased cardiovascular morbidity and mortality in ambulatory patients with chronic systolic HF,[40,41] its influence as a predictor of long-term outcomes after AHF is less well defined. The OPTIMIZE-HF registry showed that patients with DM with AHF had longer lengths of stay and increased short-term risk for rehospitalization, but similar in-hospital and short-term mortality.[39] DM was associated with increased HF rehospitalization, but not all-cause mortality in the EVEREST study.[37] However, other AHF registries have suggested that patients with DM are at increased risk for mortality.[38,42]

DM may complicate the clinical course in patients with AHF. For instance, these patients are at increased risk for adverse events during periods of reduced oral intake related to decreased appetite from congestive symptoms and NPO status for procedures. Inconsistent caloric intake along with precipitating factors for HF decompensation (eg, infection) may result in wide fluctuations in blood sugars that further perturb mental status, acid-base balance, and serum electrolytes. Long-term complications from DM, such as gastroparesis and peripheral neuropathy, may complicate AHF care by altering medication absorption, compromising nutritional status, and limiting early mobilization. Taken together, these examples highlight the importance of close attention to underlying DM and cautious management during AHF hospitalization.

There remains uncertainty in the optimal management of DM in patients with AHF. Several oral antidiabetic drugs may have harmful cardiac effects.[43,44] Thiazolidinediones (glitazones) cause sodium and water retention and may increase the risk of worsening HF.[26] Metformin initially had a relative contraindication in patients with HF when the drug was first introduced out of concern for lactic acidosis in the setting of renal impairment, but recent studies have suggested a mortality benefit.[45] Insulin use in patients with HF has been associated with increased mortality[46,47]; however, there are concerns that these findings may have been related to disease severity rather than a causal effect of the therapy itself. More recently, patients with AHF requiring insulin were found to have similar risk for adverse events after adjusting for baseline risk factors.[37] Future studies are required to explore the optimal therapeutic approach to DM during AHF hospitalization.

ANEMIA

Anemia is present in 50% to 70% of patients with HF in the ambulatory and hospital setting depending on the definition used.[48] The potential causes of anemia in patients with HF are multifactorial.[48] Patients with HF may experience an absolute or relative iron deficiency, impaired erythropoietin production caused by renal disease, reduced erythrogenesis caused by renin-angiotensin blockade, hemodilution, and anemia of chronic disease caused by the proinflammatory state. Compared with nonanemic patients with AHF, those with anemia tend to be older, with lower blood pressure and higher creatinine and natriuretic peptide levels.[49] CAD, DM, kidney disease, and COPD are more common in those with anemia.

Although a large body of data suggests that anemia is associated with worse HF outcomes,[50–52] studies have been conflicting, particularly after adjustment for baseline characteristics (eg, renal function) and disease onset and severity.[53–56] Most studies were conducted in chronic patients with HF. Thus, less is known about the outcomes of contemporary patients with AHF with baseline anemia.[55] Two recent studies have suggested that baseline anemia during AHF is associated with increased long-term morbidity and mortality.[49,57]

Despite the association between anemia and outcomes, anemia may be a prognostic marker rather than a mediator of risk. Multiple trials in chronic patients with HF, including the recent RED-HF trial,[58] investigating erythropoietin-stimulating agents have failed to demonstrate benefits on outcome.[59,60] Alternatively, the FAIR-HF trial showed that intravenous iron treatment in patients with HF with iron deficiency (with or without anemia) resulted in improved symptoms, functional capacity, and quality of life.[61] Thus, future research is needed to clarify the disconnect between the prognostic implications of anemia and the outcomes associated with treatment.

LIVER ABNORMALITIES

Abnormal liver function tests (LFTs) including aspartate transaminase (AST), alanine transaminase (ALT), alkaline phosphatase, and total bilirubin are common in patients with chronic HF[62] and patients with AHF. An analysis from EVEREST demonstrated that approximately 20% of patients with AHF have abnormalities in these laboratories.[5] The prevalence of abnormal LFTs may increase to nearly 50% in patients managed with inotropes.[63] During hospitalization, total bilirubin may be the only liver test that significantly changes; however, most of these laboratory values improve postdischarge. Studies have suggested that elevated bilirubin correlates with higher right atrial pressure and right ventricular dilation.[64] Alkaline phosphatase elevation has also been associated with marked systemic congestion and elevated right-sided filling pressure, whereas elevated AST and ALT has been associated with hypoperfusion.[63] Elevated LFTs are also associated with abnormalities in hemoglobin and natriuretic peptides.[64]

In EVEREST, elevated total bilirubin at baseline and a rise in bilirubin during hospitalization were both associated with increased morbidity and mortality. Similar findings have been demonstrated in chronic patients with HF.[62] Other studies have suggested that alkaline phosphatase and ALT and AST elevation during AHF may also be associated with increased postdischarge mortality.[63]

Abnormal LFTs are common in patients with AHF and may have prognostic relevance, but future investigation is needed to determine the implications for inpatient management. Liver dysfunction during AHF may impact drug metabolism and may further perturb other diseases, such as DM, through alterations in glucose metabolism. More significant elevations in LFTs may limit the use of medications, such as statins and amiodarone, with implications on cardiovascular comorbidities.

SLEEP APNEA

Sleep-disordered breathing (SDB) is common in patients with HF with prevalence estimates of upward of 50% to 75%.[65] Two primary types of SDB occur in patients with HF: obstructive sleep apnea (OSA) and central sleep apnea (CSA)/Cheyne-Stokes respiration. Risk factors for the development of OSA in patients with HF include male sex, elevated BMI, and increased age.[66] Lower-extremity edema has also been shown to lead to SDB, and pulmonary congestion in the setting of worsening HF further increases CSA.[67,68] Chronic SDB causes a series of derangements that may lead to the development or exacerbation of HF. SDB is proinflammatory, with nocturnal oxygen desaturations and hypercapnia seeming to play a pivotal role in the development of oxidative stress and sympathetic activation.[65] Hypertension, CAD, and DM (all well-established HF risk factors) are adversely impacted by SDB. On the other hand, HF may worsen SDB through mechanisms that include nocturnal rostral fluid movement and increased pharyngeal obstruction.[67]

The role of SDB in the clinical course, management, and outcomes of patients with AHF warrants future investigation. Untreated SDB in chronic patients with HF has been associated with increased mortality on multivariable analysis.[69] SDB has been shown to be even more common in patients with AHF than patients with chronic HF and is an independent predictor of cardiac readmission.[70,71] Observational studies assessing the efficacy of continuous positive airway pressure on morbidity and mortality in chronic patients with HF with OSA have suggested potential benefits.[65] Minute ventilation–targeted adaptive servoventilation (ASV) is a distinct form of noninvasive ventilation that automatically adjusts the degree of pressure support in response to the patient's breathing efforts. Minute ventilation–targeted ASV may treat CSA and OSA with improved tolerability compared with continuous positive airway pressure devices. Previous HF studies have demonstrated benefits on quality of life and left ventricular function with ASV[72] and randomized trials of ASV in HF are ongoing. Improved management of SDB in the AHF population may improve clinical outcomes.

CLINICAL IMPLICATIONS AND FUTURE DIRECTIONS

We have highlighted several major noncardiovascular comorbidities in patients with AHF. Other comorbidities, such as frailty, depression, nutritional deficiencies, cancer, and gout may also have direct implications on the management and outcome of patients with AHF. We have identified areas where these comorbidities may complicate HF management. In some circumstances, careful attention to the diagnosis and management of these conditions in patients with AHF may help to improve patient outcomes. As the burden of comorbidities increases in the AHF population, the potential risk for noncardiovascular adverse events increases. These considerations have implications for strategies to improve the outcomes of our patients, and also impact end point selection in clinical trials. Attention to the diagnosis and management of comorbidities represents a critical step in the holistic approach to managing patients with AHF.

REFERENCES

1. Adams KF Jr, Fonarow GC, Emerman CL, et al. Characteristics and outcomes of patients hospitalized for heart failure in the United States: rationale, design, and preliminary observations from the first 100,000 cases in the Acute Decompensated Heart Failure National Registry (ADHERE). Am Heart J 2005;149(2):209–16.
2. O'Connor CM, Abraham WT, Albert NM, et al. Predictors of mortality after discharge in patients hospitalized with heart failure: an analysis from the Organized Program to Initiate Lifesaving Treatment in Hospitalized Patients with Heart Failure (OPTIMIZE-HF). Am Heart J 2008;156(4):662–73.
3. Konstam MA, Gheorghiade M, Burnett JC Jr, et al. Effects of oral tolvaptan in patients hospitalized for worsening heart failure: the EVEREST Outcome Trial. JAMA 2007;297(12):1319–31.
4. Mentz RJ, Lewis EF. Epidemiology of cardiorenal syndrome. Heart Fail Clin 2010;6(3):333–46.
5. Ambrosy AP, Vaduganathan M, Huffman MD, et al. Clinical course and predictive value of liver function tests in patients hospitalized for worsening heart failure with reduced ejection fraction: an analysis of the EVEREST trial. Eur J Heart Fail 2012;14(3):302–11.
6. Braunstein JB, Anderson GF, Gerstenblith G, et al. Noncardiac comorbidity increases preventable hospitalizations and mortality among Medicare beneficiaries with chronic heart failure. J Am Coll Cardiol 2003;42(7):1226–33.
7. O'Connor CM, Mentz RJ, Cotter G, et al. The PROTECT in-hospital risk model: 7-day outcome in patients hospitalized with acute heart failure and renal dysfunction. Eur J Heart Fail 2012;14(6):605–12.
8. O'Connor CM, Miller AB, Blair JE, et al. Causes of death and rehospitalization in patients hospitalized

with worsening heart failure and reduced left ventricular ejection fraction: results from Efficacy of Vasopressin Antagonism in Heart Failure Outcome Study with Tolvaptan (EVEREST) program. Am Heart J 2010;159(5):841–849.e1.

9. Hawkins NM, Petrie MC, Jhund PS, et al. Heart failure and chronic obstructive pulmonary disease: diagnostic pitfalls and epidemiology. Eur J Heart Fail 2009;11(2):130–9.

10. Mentz RJ, Schulte PJ, Fleg JL, et al. Clinical characteristics, response to exercise training, and outcomes in patients with heart failure and chronic obstructive pulmonary disease: findings from Heart Failure and A Controlled Trial Investigating Outcomes of Exercise TraiNing (HF-ACTION). Am Heart J 2013;165(2):193–9.

11. Dahlstrom U. Frequent non-cardiac comorbidities in patients with chronic heart failure. Eur J Heart Fail 2005;7(3):309–16.

12. Mentz RJ, Fiuzat M, Wojdyla DM, et al. Clinical characteristics and outcomes of hospitalized heart failure patients with systolic dysfunction and chronic obstructive pulmonary disease: findings from OPTIMIZE-HF. Eur J Heart Fail 2012;14(4): 395–403.

13. Mentz RJ, Schmidt PH, Kwasny MJ, et al. The impact of chronic obstructive pulmonary disease in patients hospitalized for worsening heart failure with reduced ejection fraction: an analysis of the EVEREST Trial. J Card Fail 2012;18(7): 515–23.

14. Hawkins NM, Petrie MC, Macdonald MR, et al. Heart failure and chronic obstructive pulmonary disease the quandary of beta-blockers and beta-agonists. J Am Coll Cardiol 2011;57(21): 2127–38.

15. Dungen HD, Apostolovic S, Inkrot S, et al. Titration to target dose of bisoprolol vs. carvedilol in elderly patients with heart failure: the CIBIS-ELD trial. Eur J Heart Fail 2011;13(6):670–80.

16. Mentz RJ, Fiuzat M, Kraft M, et al. Bronchodilators in heart failure patients with COPD: is it time for a clinical trial? J Card Fail 2012;18(5):413–22.

17. Salpeter S, Ormiston T, Salpeter E. Cardioselective beta-blockers for chronic obstructive pulmonary disease. Cochrane Database Syst Rev 2005;(4): CD003566.

18. Mentz RJ, Wojdyla D, Fiuzat M, et al. Association of beta-blocker use and selectivity with outcomes in patients with heart failure and chronic obstructive pulmonary disease (from OPTIMIZE-HF). Am J Cardiol 2013;111(4):582–7.

19. Ronco C, Haapio M, House AA, et al. Cardiorenal syndrome. J Am Coll Cardiol 2008;52(19):1527–39.

20. Blair JE, Pang PS, Schrier RW, et al. Changes in renal function during hospitalization and soon after discharge in patients admitted for worsening heart failure in the placebo group of the EVEREST trial. Eur Heart J 2011;32(20):2563–72.

21. Hillege HL, Nitsch D, Pfeffer MA, et al. Renal function as a predictor of outcome in a broad spectrum of patients with heart failure. Circulation 2006; 113(5):671–8.

22. Dries DL, Exner DV, Domanski MJ, et al. The prognostic implications of renal insufficiency in asymptomatic and symptomatic patients with left ventricular systolic dysfunction. J Am Coll Cardiol 2000;35(3):681–9.

23. Heywood JT, Fonarow GC, Costanzo MR, et al. High prevalence of renal dysfunction and its impact on outcome in 118,465 patients hospitalized with acute decompensated heart failure: a report from the ADHERE database. J Card Fail 2007;13(6):422–30.

24. Butler J, Forman DE, Abraham WT, et al. Relationship between heart failure treatment and development of worsening renal function among hospitalized patients. Am Heart J 2004;147(2): 331–8.

25. Jose P, Skali H, Anavekar N, et al. Increase in creatinine and cardiovascular risk in patients with systolic dysfunction after myocardial infarction. J Am Soc Nephrol 2006;17(10):2886–91.

26. McMurray JJ, Adamopoulos S, Anker SD, et al. ESC Guidelines for the diagnosis and treatment of acute and chronic heart failure 2012: the Task Force for the Diagnosis and Treatment of Acute and Chronic Heart Failure 2012 of the European Society of Cardiology. Developed in collaboration with the Heart Failure Association (HFA) of the ESC. Eur Heart J 2012;33(14):1787–847.

27. McMurray J, Cohen-Solal A, Dietz R, et al. Practical recommendations for the use of ACE inhibitors, beta-blockers, aldosterone antagonists and angiotensin receptor blockers in heart failure: putting guidelines into practice. Eur J Heart Fail 2005; 7(5):710–21.

28. Felker GM, Mentz RJ. Diuretics and ultrafiltration in acute decompensated heart failure. J Am Coll Cardiol 2012;59(24):2145–53.

29. Damman K, Navis G, Voors AA, et al. Worsening renal function and prognosis in heart failure: systematic review and meta-analysis. J Card Fail 2007;13(8):599–608.

30. Owan TE, Hodge DO, Herges RM, et al. Secular trends in renal dysfunction and outcomes in hospitalized heart failure patients. J Card Fail 2006; 12(4):257–62.

31. Smith GL, Vaccarino V, Kosiborod M, et al. Worsening renal function: what is a clinically meaningful change in creatinine during hospitalization with heart failure? J Card Fail 2003;9(1):13–25.

32. Forman DE, Butler J, Wang Y, et al. Incidence, predictors at admission, and impact of worsening

renal function among patients hospitalized with heart failure. J Am Coll Cardiol 2004;43(1):61–7.

33. Aronson D, Burger AJ. The relationship between transient and persistent worsening renal function and mortality in patients with acute decompensated heart failure. J Card Fail 2010;16(7):541–7.

34. Testani JM, Chen J, McCauley BD, et al. Potential effects of aggressive decongestion during the treatment of decompensated heart failure on renal function and survival. Circulation 2010;122(3):265–72.

35. Felker GM, Lee KL, Bull DA, et al. Diuretic strategies in patients with acute decompensated heart failure. N Engl J Med 2011;364(9):797–805.

36. Stevenson LW, Zile M, Bennett TD, et al. Chronic ambulatory intracardiac pressures and future heart failure events. Circ Heart Fail 2010;3(5):580–7.

37. Sarma S, Mentz RJ, Kwasny MJ, et al. Association between diabetes mellitus and post-discharge outcomes in patients hospitalized with heart failure: findings from the EVEREST trial. Eur J Heart Fail 2013;15(2):194–202.

38. Parissis JT, Rafouli-Stergiou P, Mebazaa A, et al. Acute heart failure in patients with diabetes mellitus: clinical characteristics and predictors of in-hospital mortality. Int J Cardiol 2012;157(1): 108–13.

39. Greenberg BH, Abraham WT, Albert NM, et al. Influence of diabetes on characteristics and outcomes in patients hospitalized with heart failure: a report from the Organized Program to Initiate Lifesaving Treatment in Hospitalized Patients with Heart Failure (OPTIMIZE-HF). Am Heart J 2007; 154(2):277.e1–8.

40. MacDonald MR, Petrie MC, Varyani F, et al. Impact of diabetes on outcomes in patients with low and preserved ejection fraction heart failure: an analysis of the Candesartan in Heart failure: Assessment of Reduction in Mortality and morbidity (CHARM) programme. Eur Heart J 2008;29(11): 1377–85.

41. De Groote P, Lamblin N, Mouquet F, et al. Impact of diabetes mellitus on long-term survival in patients with congestive heart failure. Eur Heart J 2004; 25(8):656–62.

42. Harjola VP, Follath F, Nieminen MS, et al. Characteristics, outcomes, and predictors of mortality at 3 months and 1 year in patients hospitalized for acute heart failure. Eur J Heart Fail 2010;12(3): 239–48.

43. Schramm TK, Gislason GH, Vaag A, et al. Mortality and cardiovascular risk associated with different insulin secretagogues compared with metformin in type 2 diabetes, with or without a previous myocardial infarction: a nationwide study. Eur Heart J 2011;32(15):1900–8.

44. Nissen SE, Wolski K. Rosiglitazone revisited: an updated meta-analysis of risk for myocardial infarction and cardiovascular mortality. Arch Intern Med 2010;170(14):1191–201.

45. MacDonald MR, Eurich DT, Majumdar SR, et al. Treatment of type 2 diabetes and outcomes in patients with heart failure: a nested case-control study from the U.K. General Practice Research Database. Diabetes Care 2010;33(6): 1213–8.

46. Smooke S, Horwich TB, Fonarow GC. Insulin-treated diabetes is associated with a marked increase in mortality in patients with advanced heart failure. Am Heart J 2005;149(1):168–74.

47. Murcia AM, Hennekens CH, Lamas GA, et al. Impact of diabetes on mortality in patients with myocardial infarction and left ventricular dysfunction. Arch Intern Med 2004;164(20):2273–9.

48. Anand IS. Anemia and chronic heart failure implications and treatment options. J Am Coll Cardiol 2008;52(7):501–11.

49. von Haehling S, Schefold JC, Hodoscek LM, et al. Anaemia is an independent predictor of death in patients hospitalized for acute heart failure. Clin Res Cardiol 2010;99(2):107–13.

50. Lindenfeld J. Prevalence of anemia and effects on mortality in patients with heart failure. Am Heart J 2005;149(3):391–401.

51. Groenveld HF, Januzzi JL, Damman K, et al. Anemia and mortality in heart failure patients a systematic review and meta-analysis. J Am Coll Cardiol 2008;52(10):818–27.

52. Tang YD, Katz SD. The prevalence of anemia in chronic heart failure and its impact on the clinical outcomes. Heart Fail Rev 2008;13(4):387–92.

53. Kosiborod M, Curtis JP, Wang Y, et al. Anemia and outcomes in patients with heart failure: a study from the National Heart Care Project. Arch Intern Med 2005;165(19):2237–44.

54. Maraldi C, Volpato S, Cesari M, et al. Anemia, physical disability, and survival in older patients with heart failure. J Card Fail 2006;12(7):533–9.

55. Felker GM, Gattis WA, Leimberger JD, et al. Usefulness of anemia as a predictor of death and rehospitalization in patients with decompensated heart failure. Am J Cardiol 2003;92(5):625–8.

56. Kalra PR, Collier T, Cowie MR, et al. Haemoglobin concentration and prognosis in new cases of heart failure. Lancet 2003;362(9379):211–2.

57. Hamaguchi S, Tsuchihashi-Makaya M, Kinugawa S, et al. Anemia is an independent predictor of long-term adverse outcomes in patients hospitalized with heart failure in Japan. A report from the Japanese Cardiac Registry of Heart Failure in Cardiology (JCARE-CARD). Circ J 2009; 73(10):1901–8.

58. Swedberg K, Young JB, Anand IS, et al. Treatment of anemia with darbepoetin alfa in systolic heart failure. N Engl J Med 2013;368(13):1210–9.

59. van Veldhuisen DJ, Dickstein K, Cohen-Solal A, et al. Randomized, double-blind, placebo-controlled study to evaluate the effect of two dosing regimens of darbepoetin alfa in patients with heart failure and anaemia. Eur Heart J 2007; 28(18):2208–16.

60. Ghali JK, Anand IS, Abraham WT, et al. Randomized double-blind trial of darbepoetin alfa in patients with symptomatic heart failure and anemia. Circulation 2008;117(4):526–35.

61. Anker SD, Comin Colet J, Filippatos G, et al. Ferric carboxymaltose in patients with heart failure and iron deficiency. N Engl J Med 2009;361(25): 2436–48.

62. Allen LA, Felker GM, Pocock S, et al. Liver function abnormalities and outcome in patients with chronic heart failure: data from the Candesartan in Heart Failure: Assessment of Reduction in Mortality and Morbidity (CHARM) program. Eur J Heart Fail 2009;11(2):170–7.

63. Nikolaou M, Parissis J, Yilmaz MB, et al. Liver function abnormalities, clinical profile, and outcome in acute decompensated heart failure. Eur Heart J 2013;34(10):742–9.

64. Biegus J, Zymlinski R, Sokolski M, et al. Liver function tests in patients with acute heart failure. Pol Arch Med Wewn 2012;122(10):471–9.

65. Kasai T, Bradley TD. Obstructive sleep apnea and heart failure: pathophysiologic and therapeutic implications. J Am Coll Cardiol 2011;57(2):119–27.

66. Bradley TD, Floras JS. Sleep apnea and heart failure. Part I: obstructive sleep apnea. Circulation 2003;107(12):1671–8.

67. Yumino D, Redolfi S, Ruttanaumpawan P, et al. Nocturnal rostral fluid shift: a unifying concept for the pathogenesis of obstructive and central sleep apnea in men with heart failure. Circulation 2010; 121(14):1598–605.

68. Solin P, Bergin P, Richardson M, et al. Influence of pulmonary capillary wedge pressure on central apnea in heart failure. Circulation 1999;99(12): 1574–9.

69. Wang H, Parker JD, Newton GE, et al. Influence of obstructive sleep apnea on mortality in patients with heart failure. J Am Coll Cardiol 2007;49(15): 1625–31.

70. Khayat RN, Jarjoura D, Patt B, et al. In-hospital testing for sleep-disordered breathing in hospitalized patients with decompensated heart failure: report of prevalence and patient characteristics. J Card Fail 2009;15(9):739–46.

71. Khayat R, Abraham W, Patt B, et al. Central sleep apnea is a predictor of cardiac readmission in hospitalized patients with systolic heart failure. J Card Fail 2012;18(7):534–40.

72. Sharma BK, Bakker JP, McSharry DG, et al. Adaptive servoventilation for treatment of sleep-disordered breathing in heart failure: a systematic review and meta-analysis. Chest 2012;142(5): 1211–21.

Index

Note: Page numbers of article titles are in **boldface** type.

Heart Failure Clin 9 (2013) 369–371
http://dx.doi.org/10.1016/S1551-7136(13)00039-1
1551-7136/13/$ – see front matter © 2013 Elsevier Inc. All rights reserved.

heartfailure.theclinics.com

Moving?

Make sure your subscription moves with you!

To notify us of your new address, find your **Clinics Account Number** (located on your mailing label above your name), and contact customer service at:

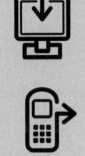

Email: journalscustomerservice-usa@elsevier.com

800-654-2452 (subscribers in the U.S. & Canada)
314-447-8871 (subscribers outside of the U.S. & Canada)

Fax number: 314-447-8029

Elsevier Health Sciences Division
Subscription Customer Service
3251 Riverport Lane
Maryland Heights, MO 63043

*To ensure uninterrupted delivery of your subscription, please notify us at least 4 weeks in advance of move.

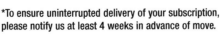

Moving?

Make sure your subscription moves with you!

Printed and bound by CPI Group (UK) Ltd, Croydon, CR0 4YY

03/10/2024

01040332-0011